Mrs B Pickering
ECG.

Manual of Echocardiographic Techniques

BETTY J. PHILLIPS, R.D.M.S.

Chief Ultrasound Technologist
Supervisor of Education
Ultrasound Diagnostic Services, Ltd.
Phoenix, Arizona

with the assistance of

VINCENT E. FRIEDEWALD, Jr., M.D., F.A.C.C., F.A.C.P.

Chief of Cardiology, The Honolulu Medical Group, Inc.
Assistant Clinical Professor of Medicine,
John A. Burns School of Medicine,
University of Hawaii, Honolulu, Hawaii

1980
W. B. SAUNDERS COMPANY
Philadelphia   London   Toronto

W. B. Saunders Company: West Washington Square
Philadelphia, PA   19105

1 St. Anne's Road
Eastbourne, East Sussex BN21 3UN, England

1 Goldthorne Avenue
Toronto, Ontario M8Z 5T9, Canada

Library of Congress Cataloging in Publication Data

Phillips, Betty J
    Manual of echocardiographic techniques.

    1. Ultrasonic cardiography.   2. Heart — Diseases — Diagnosis.
I. Friedewald, Vincent E., joint author.
II. Title. [DNLM: 1. Echocardiography — Methods.
WG141.5.E2 P558m]
RC683.5.U5P48   616.1′2′0754   79-3921

ISBN 0-7216-7219-1

Manual of Echocardiographic Techniques   ISBN   0-7216-7219-1

Last digit is the print number: 9   8   7   6   5   4   3   2   1

TO MY MOTHER
AND
IN MEMORY OF MY FATHER

FOREWORD

The quality of the M-mode echocardiogram is more dependent on the ability of the individual performing the test than on any other factor. Unfortunately, failure to recognize the importance of the echo technologist's skill and underestimation of the time and effort required to attain that skill remain critical barriers to the universal attainment of excellence in cardiac ultrasound. The *Manual of Echocardiographic Techniques* is adequate testimony to the magnitude of knowledge that must be learned before this level of competence can be achieved.

Ms. Betty Phillips is one of the pioneers among those responsible for today's rapidly advancing state of the art. In clinical and research laboratories in the early 1970's, she was one of the first to demonstrate that both misuse of instrumentation and incorrect transducer angle were important causes of false-positive and false-negative diagnoses. Yet, although almost 10 years later the lessons we learned then about transducer angle and instrument control are more important than ever, they still remain sadly neglected in the literature.

In the *Manual of Echocardiographic Techniques*, Ms. Phillips presents the technical intricacies of performing an echocardiogram both by means of the written text and by carefully selected illustrations of tracings. However, she leaves no question that technique alone does not suffice in her discussions of cardiac anatomy and the disease processes that affect cardiac structure and function.

Finally, although the importance of technique and knowledge of cardiac anatomy and pathology cannot be overemphasized, Ms. Phillips so rightly presents an additional dimension in the technologist's approach to her task. This dimension is the human aspect alluded to, for example, in her discussion of patient comfort. We should always remember that an echocardiogram does not represent simply a cold interaction between man and machine but also a meeting between two human beings, a fact so often forgotten in our age of ever-increasing technology.

VINCENT E. FRIEDEWALD, JR., M.D.
Honolulu, Hawaii

PREFACE

This volume is intended as a textbook for the student of adult echocardiography and as a practical reference handbook for the physician utilizing echocardiography for clinical medicine and for practicing sonographers who wish to further their knowledge of this technique. It presents the techniques of conducting the echocardiographic examination to produce accurate images and methods of interpretation necessary to evaluate the quality of those images.

The sequence of chapters is deliberate. Each topic is dependent upon the one that precedes it, and the order is that which I have found best suited to guide the reader to a solid understanding of the basic techniques of the echocardiographic examination and its important pitfalls.

Repetition is freely used whenever it is felt necessary to emphasize important topics, especially in overlapping areas or in different contexts.

Chapter 1 provides the reader with the basic concepts and physical properties that constitute the ultrasound principle. Chapter 2 presents a detailed account of all that is involved in performing the echocardiographic examination, and Chapter 3 demonstrates in detail the value of recording a simultaneous electrocardiogram. Chapters 4 through 12 deal with the echocardiographic technique of recording the various cardiac structures. Each of these chapters demonstrates the anatomy of these structures, familiarizing the reader with the many variations of normal and pathological conditions and how these variations appear on the echocardiogram.

To these ends, this book emphasizes the technical and diagnostic aspects of adult M-mode echocardiography, leaving a discussion of its research uses to others in the field of investigation.

BETTY J. PHILLIPS, R.D.M.S.
Phoenix, Arizona

ACKNOWLEDGMENTS

Leading all acknowledgments must be mine to Jacklyn L. Ellis, M.A., R.D.M.S., my associate and friend, who in addition to having performed a masterful job of writing what in my opinion was the most difficult chapter (Chapter 12 — Prosthetic Valves), was also an invaluable participant throughout the entire writing of this book. Her unfaltering support and assistance in resolving the countless details that are encountered in such an endeavor has truly made this book possible.

Also, my deep gratitude goes to:

Vincent E. Friedewald, Jr., M.D., my teacher and friend, who inspired the need for such a book and spent innumerable hours in reviewing, refining, and correcting the manuscript with a reassuring respect for accuracy. Whatever success this book earns, I share with him.

Karen A. Keeton, a good friend and the artist who is responsible for the excellent illustrations of the heart. I am most grateful to Ms. Keeton not only for her outstanding drawings but also for her enthusiastic cooperation, innovative ideas, and total dedication to never settling for less than perfection.

David Sansbury, Biomedical Engineer, St. Joseph's Hospital and Medical Center, for his collaboration with me in the presentation on the physics of ultrasound in Chapter 1.

I would also like to express my appreciation to Edward B. Diethrich, M.D., the Arizona Heart Institute, and St. Joseph's Hospital and Medical Center, who made many of the studies described in this text possible.

I do not really know how to thank my co-workers at Ultrasound Diagnostic Services for their patience with what seemed at times like a ramshackle and never-ending project. My thanks to them for never saying so, and for their indefatigable good spirits.

Lastly, I would like to gratefully acknowledge the wholehearted cooperation of the W. B. Saunders Company in the production of this book, with special thanks to Jack Hanley who believed in it from the beginning and to Wendy Phillips for her positive attitude and tenacity in keeping open the lines of communication.

BETTY J. PHILLIPS, R.D.M.S.

CONTENTS

Chapter 1

PHYSICAL PROPERTIES OF ULTRASOUND

Although it is not necessary for the technologist to deal with the physical principles of ultrasonic energy in a quantitative sense, i.e., with numerical values and formulae, an understanding of the qualitative or behavioral aspects of this type of energy is essential. Knowledge of how it is produced, how it behaves, and how it can be employed in the clinical setting is fundamental to developing the techniques and judgments that yield useful diagnostic information.

Inasmuch as the character of ultrasound is paramount in this discussion, a rigorous treatment of its physical principles will not be attempted. In fact, it may be useful at times to simplify the concept by thinking of ultrasound as something in between the light and sound energy familiar to our senses. An excellent analysis of the subject has been provided by Wells.[1]

The goal here is to provide the technologist with an understanding of how ultrasonic energy is generated, what happens to it as it traverses the biological medium, why it is reflected, how it is detected, and how it may be used in diagnostic ultrasound.

DIAGNOSTIC ULTRASOUND SYSTEMS

There are two types of ultrasound that are useful in clinical medicine, the Doppler system and the pulse-echo system. In both types, ultrasonic energy is generated by a transmitting transducer* that is placed in physical contact with the biological medium (body tissue).

Transmitted energy enters and traverses the body tissue until it encounters a reflective component (an organ or skeletal member). At the point of encounter, a portion of the transmitted energy is reflected back to a receiving transducer. The balance of the transmitted energy may subsequently encounter other reflective components, giving rise to additional transmitted and reflected signals (Fig. 1–1). Reflected energy returns through the biological medium until it reaches the point at which it is sensed (detected) by a receiving transducer. The ultrasonic energy of both the Doppler and the pulse-echo systems behaves in this manner. The two techniques differ primarily in the way in which the transducers are excited and in the means used to process the return information. (Fig. 1–2).

Doppler Ultrasound

With Doppler ultrasound, the transmitter is continuously excited with a single high

---

*A transducer, in the broad sense, is any device that converts energy from one form to another. The ultrasound transducer converts electrical energy to ultrasonic energy (transmitting transducer), or it converts ultrasonic energy into electrical energy (receiving transducer). The transmitter and the receiver may be the same device or two separate instruments.

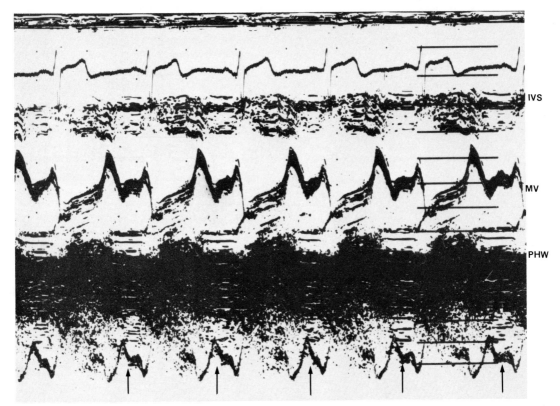

IVS

MV

PHW

Figure 1–1. Reflections. Sound waves can be reflected more than once before returning to the transducer. In this M-mode recording of the mitral valve (MV), an inverted image of the mitral valve (arrows) is seen behind the posterior heart wall (PHW). This is not an uncommon occurrence in thin-chested individuals, as some of the returning echoes from the mitral valve are reflected off two other structures, such as the chest wall and sternum, before returning to the transducer (IVS = interventricular septum).

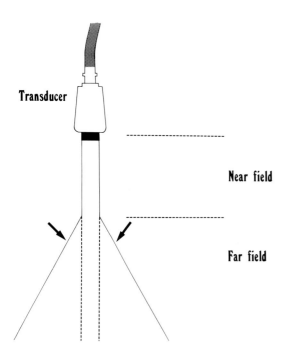

Transducer

Near field

Far field

Figure 1–2. The sound beam. In the near field, the beam width remains equal to the diameter of the transducer. In the far field, beam divergence occurs (arrows).

frequency. The frequency of the returned energy differs from the frequency of the transmitted energy, and that difference is proportional to the velocity of the reflecting component encountered. In clinical practice, the reflecting component is most commonly blood flowing in arteries or veins, so the frequency change (Doppler shift) is indicative of blood velocity. Since the transmitting transducer is continuously generating ultrasonic energy, it is common to employ a second transducer as a receiver.

Pulse-Echo Ultrasound

With pulse-echo ultrasound, the transducer is excited at intervals, and energy is transmitted in short bursts. Since the speed of ultrasonic energy is relatively uniform in biological tissue, the time elapsed from transmission of the burst (pulse) to reception of the reflection (echo) is representative of the distance between the transducer and

the reflective component (Fig. 1–3). Since the transducer is transmitting only in bursts, the same device can be used for receiving the echo. Thus, it is common to employ only a single transducer with pulse-echo ultrasound. Less than one half of 1/100 of one second is required for the generation, transmission, reflection, and return of ultrasonic energy. Therefore, it is possible to apply the pulse-echo sequence (energy generation, transmission, reflection, echo detection) frequently, thus determining the position of an internal organ with time.

In practice, the equipment is designed to produce approximately one pulse-echo sequence per millisecond. Velocity as well as positional information are therefore available with pulse-echo ultrasound. For example, suppose that the elapsed time of a pulse-echo sequence indicated the position of a mitral valve leaflet to be 8.20 cm from the transducer (skin surface). Suppose that the elapsed time of the pulse-echo sequence one millisecond later indicated the

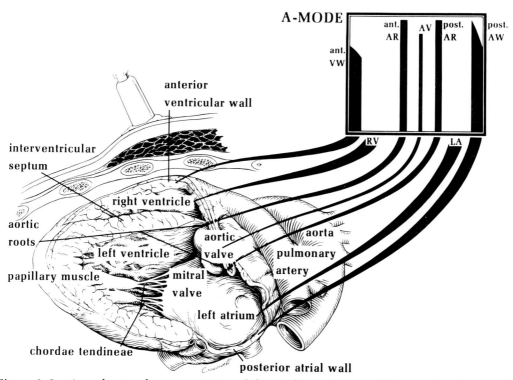

Figure 1–3. A-mode signal representation of the cardiac structures. Ultrasound echoes are displayed on the oscilloscope as individual peaks directly related to their anatomical location and their reflector strength. Key: Ant. VW = anterior ventricular wall; RV = right ventricle; Ant. AR = anterior aortic root; AV = aortic valve; Post. AR = posterior aortic root; LA = left atrium; Post. AW = posterior anterior wall.

same leaflet to be 8.24 cm from the transducer. The positional change from 8.20 cm to 8.24 = 0.04 cm, which divided by the time interval between pulses (0.001 sec) yields the velocity (40 cm per sec). The fact that the leaflet was more distant during the second pulse-echo sequence indicates the direction of motion to be away from the transducer (mitral valve closing).

GENERATION OF ULTRASONIC ENERGY

Although it is beyond the range of human hearing, ultrasonic energy is sound energy in the true sense, and it is generated in much the same way as audible sound. In essence, a structure in mechanical vibration establishes regions of compression and rarefaction in the medium that it contacts. The speaker of a radio, for example, vibrates and creates sound energy in the air surrounding it. Ultrasonic energy is generated in precisely the same manner, but at a much higher vibratory rate. While vibrating cycles for audible sound occur from 30 to 15,000 times per second, medically useful ultrasound employs vibratory cycles occurring from two to five million times per second. It is primarily this higher frequency of vibration that causes the behavioral difference between ultrasound and audible sound. The structure establishing vibration is termed the sound source and is usually a transducer.

ULTRASOUND TRANSDUCERS

The speaker of a radio is an audio-sound transducer. It converts electrical energy, via vibratory motion, into sound energy. While not normally used as such, a radio speaker can also convert vibratory motion into electrical energy. The mass and size of a radio speaker prohibit vibrations much beyond 20 thousand cycles per second (20 kHz).

The high frequencies of ultrasound are produced by piezoelectric crystals, which form the basis of all ultrasound transducers. The piezoelectric effect is the unique quality of a material to deform under the influence of electrical excitations or, likewise, to create electrical signals when it is mechanically deformed. Quartz crystals have this quality, but the substance most commonly used in medical applications is the synthetic piezoelectric material PZT (lead-zirconate-titanate). For use in a transducer, both sides of a PZT disc are coated with metal (usually silver), which is then connected with the electronic equipment. When an electrical potential is created between the two metal layers, the piezoelectric disc deforms, causing its center to "bulge" out of the plane of the periphery (as the diaphragm of a drum). The direction of the bulge is determined by the polarity of the electrical potential, and the extent of the bulge is determined by the magnitude. It is easy to see, then, that when the disc is placed in contact with the skin, electrical potentials can be applied to the metal layers

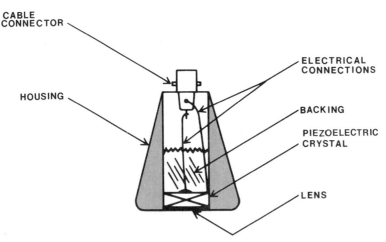

CABLE CONNECTOR

HOUSING

ELECTRICAL CONNECTIONS

BACKING

PIEZOELECTRIC CRYSTAL

LENS

Figure 1–4. The ultrasound transducer. The principal element of the transducer is a disc of piezoelectric ceramic positioned immediately behind the lens. The piezoelectric crystal has the innate double property of (1) producing ultrasonic pulses from voltages applied to it through the electrical connections from the machine cable and (2) converting the returning ultrasound pulses to electrical impulses that represent the echo on the oscilloscope (see Figure 1–3).

The sound waves generated back into the transducer are absorbed by an insulating material within the transducer housing.

either to push against the skin or to pull away from it. In practice, a metal-coated piezoelectric disc is mounted on a plastic material through which the ultrasound vibrations are conveyed to the skin. This is done to electrically isolate and mechanically protect the fragile piezoelectric disc. The disc and the plastic sound conductor are encased in a structure that is easily held and that provides strain relief for the electrical wires leading to the energy source. While it has numerous mechanical characteristics, the ultrasound transducer is essentially a metal-coated piezoelectric disc with a plastic rod connecting it acoustically to the medium, electrical wires connecting the metal coatings to the energy source, and a casing designed for protection and ease of handling. The basic structure of a pulse-echo ultrasound transducer is shown in Figure 1–4.

The vibrations of a radio speaker, particularly at low frequency, can be seen and felt. As the vibrations increase in frequency, the speaker diaphragm motion is less perceptible because the excursions are shorter and more rapid. The vibrations of the piezoelectric material are imperceptible to the human senses because the excursions are many times smaller than in a radio speaker. Nevertheless, the action is essentially the same.

NATURE OF ULTRASONIC ENERGY

The pushing and pulling of the transducer against the biological medium sets up disturbances called regions of compression and rarefaction. Since cells of tissue are interconnected, the disturbances (vibrations) are transferred through the tissue, and, at each point along the path, the vibratory motions are the same as those experienced by the transmitting transducer. That some internal point is set into vibratory motion is evidence that energy is entering and traversing the medium. Ultrasonic energy travels by wave motion and is governed by the applicable physical principles.

Velocity

The velocity of ultrasonic energy is controlled by the medium through which it travels. In biological material, for example, ultrasonic energy travels at an approximate velocity of 1500 meters per second (M/sec). While the material itself does not experience any net motion, the position of a compressive disturbance will change. An analogy can be drawn to the toy intercom made of tin cans and a string. The string does not experience any net motion, but energy obviously travels through the string from tin can to tin can. The concepts of importance are (1) that ultrasound energy travels through a medium without the medium experiencing net motion and (2) that the velocity of travel is dependent solely on the qualities of the medium.

The Ultrasound Beam

Unlike the sound energy from a radio speaker, ultrasonic energy does not travel away from its source in all directions. It travels more like a beam of light, and only a slight beam spreading (divergence) is exhibited (see Figure 1–2). This "beam" quality of ultrasonic energy derives from the relative dimensions of the source (transducer) and the wavelength of the ultrasound. Since wavelength is inversely related to frequency, the very high frequencies of ultrasound are accompanied by very short wavelengths. A wavelength can be imagined as the distance between adjacent regions in compressive disturbance. Obviously, the time between adjacent compressive regions is determined by the vibratory frequency of the transducer.

If the velocity with which the disturbance travels away from the transducer is known, then the distance between adjacent disturbances can be determined. Suppose a piezoelectric disc with a diameter of 1 cm were used to generate sound or ultrasonic energy. With the disc vibrating at 1000 Hz, the resulting wavelength in the biological tissue would be 200 cm — 2000 times the source dimension, and significant divergence could be expected. At 2000 Hz, however, the wavelength would be only 1 mm, or 0.1 of the source dimension, and little beam divergence would result.

Just as a beam of light can be focused, the ultrasound beam can be concentrated. This is accomplished by forming a concave surface in the sound-coupling material of the transducer where it contacts the skin. The important concept here is that the high frequencies of ultrasound mitigate energy spreading (or divergence), so that ultrasonic energy travels through the medium as a beam.

Resolution

Generation of an energy "beam" is not the only reason for employing high-frequency ultrasound as a diagnostic tool. As previously stated, a portion of the transmitting energy is reflected and returned to the transducer, where it is processed to provide positional information. Physical contraints dictate that a sizable portion of the returned energy wavelength be received simply to identify its presence. A sizable portion of the 22-cm wavelength of a 1000-Hz signal might represent 40 cm of distance and would not provide useful information. Knowing the position of an internal organ within 0.2 of the 1-mm wavelength of a 2-MHz signal, however, is significant. As a general observation, then, the high frequencies of ultrasound are commensurate with higher resolution (positional certainty).

Attenuation

If it is true that higher frequency is accompanied by low ultrasound beam divergence and high resolution, then why not use frequencies even higher than the 2 to 4 MHz commonly employed? The reason for limiting the frequency is to reduce attenuation. As ultrasonic energy travels through the body, it is absorbed and scattered by minute surfaces. Because the degree of absorption and scattering is proportional to frequency, an increase in ultrasound frequency will increase the attenuation.

The overall attenuation also depends on the distance that the ultrasonic energy travels entering and returning from the body. Attenuation combined with the fact that only a small portion of incident energy is reflected from internal organs results in an exceedingly faint echo at the receiving transducer. At 2.5 MHz, echoes from organs

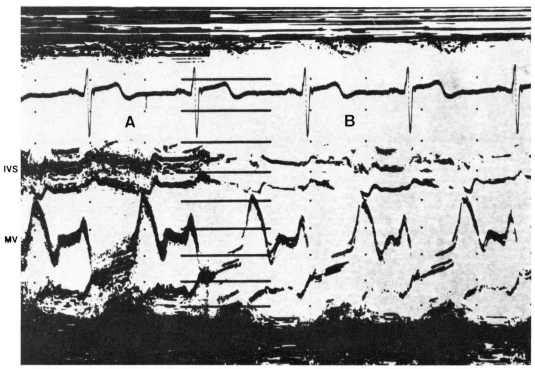

Figure 1–5. The near gain control (not visible) is properly positioned in the area designated A during the first two beats; as a result, the full interventricular septum (IVS) and the mitral valve leaflets (MV) are clearly seen. In the area designated B, following the second beat, the delay (attenuation) is incorrectly adjusted, and the septum and mitral valve leaflets are poorly visualized.

proximal to the transducer may return only 0.25 per cent of the transmitted energy.

Since echoes from distal surfaces are many times smaller than echoes from proximal reflection sites, greater amplification is required for distal echoes. Commercially available ultrasound instruments provide a time-gain control for this purpose. Since distal echoes occur later in time, the technologist may select the amplification that will produce the most meaningful information. Such controls normally provide for selecting both the time at which the amplification increase will start after each ultrasonic energy burst and the rate of increase once amplification increase has commenced. If, for example, the internal structure of interest lies between 5 cm and 12 cm below the body surface, the technologist would set the amplification increase to begin at a time representing 5 cm. The rate of amplification increase would then be selected so that echoes from the 12 cm surface would be intelligibly amplified. Echoes from beyond the 12 cm depth, then, would not be pronounced, owing to attenuation. While the time-gain controls are conceptually quite simple, they provide the technologist with a powerful tool for eliciting the desired information (Fig. 1–5).

Reflections

The various components of the body (tissue, muscle, bone, blood, and so on) have a property called acoustic, or characteristic, impedance. Although the property is a measure of the components' ability to conduct ultrasound waves, it is sufficient here to understand its relationship to echoes (reflections). When an ultrasound beam encounters the surface between two media of different characteristic impedances, a portion of the incidental energy is reflected from the interface surface back into the first medium, and the balance enters the second medium (see Figure 1–1). The amount of energy reflected depends on the difference in the characteristic impedances. The portion of incident energy reflected from the interface surface increases as the difference in characteristic impedance between the two media increases. Except for bone, most biological materials have nearly equal characteristic impedance. For this reason, echoes from an interface surface are generally small. For example, the surface between the heart and the blood reflects only about 1 per cent of the incident energy. Bone, however, has a very high characteristic impedance, as does air. A muscle-bone interface reflects nearly 50 per cent of the incident energy. This is the fundamental reason that the intercostal spaces must be used to view the heart — otherwise, the rib bones would return most of the energy immediately to the transducer and impede any echoes that did derive from the heart itself. Several biological components, in order of increasing characteristic impedance, are: fat, brain, blood, kidney, tissue, spleen, liver, muscle, and bone. A stronger echo would be expected from the fat-epicardium interface than from the endocardium-blood interface just beyond. Echoes do not occur without a homogeneous material. Therefore, no echoes would be expected from the area between the epicardial and endocardial surfaces.

As with light, the angle of reflection and the angle of incidence of the ultrasound beam are equal. In practice, however, it is not necessary to have the ultrasound beam strike a surface at right angles. While the echo will be stronger with orthogonal incidence, surfaces are sufficiently rough to reflect some energy back to the transducer. To derive the best echo from the surface of interest, the technologist may compromise orthogonal incidence for beam path length.

REFERENCE

1. Wells PNT: *Physical Principles of Ultrasonic Diagnosis.* New York, Academic Press, 1969.

Chapter 2

THE ECHOCARDIOGRAPHIC EXAMINATION

Most patients approach any type of medical test with some degree of apprehension. Even an individual who feels certain that he is healthy may be concerned, particularly when he is undergoing a test that is not familiar to him. A great deal of strain can be relieved if the technologist simply presents a confident and friendly appearance.

For the patient who has never had an echocardiogram, the basic procedure should be explained, emphasizing that the examination is safe and painless and that the knowledge gained from the test will assist the physician in the evaluation of the patient's heart. It is also advisable that the technologist explain that this information will be taken from a graphic recording (not an actual picture of the heart), which is carefully measured and interpreted by a physician. By informing the patient of such details, the technologist will gain his confidence and interest and will facilitate the performance of the examination.

A further consideration is the patient's modesty, which is particularly important for the female patient. The examiner should leave the room while the patient is changing for the examination or provide a screened changing area. A hospital gown worn with the opening in the front will afford the technologist sufficient space in which to position the transducer and still maintain the patient's modesty.

Some patients, especially elderly persons, become easily chilled. It is therefore a good practice to keep either an extra sheet or a blanket at hand, as warmth is essential to relaxation.

Finally, the attitude of the technologist can also have a significant effect on the quality of the echocardiographic examination. A positive, confident approach to even the most difficult situation will reduce tension and can contribute significantly to the successful performance of the examination.

PATIENT POSITIONING

Technically superior recordings are most often obtained with the patient positioned on his left side. When this position is not possible, the patient should lie supine. In either position, the patient should be encouraged to make himself as comfortable as possible. When the patient is comfortable, he will not tire as easily, and the incidence of echocardiographic artifact due to muscle tension will be lessened (Fig. 2–1).

OBSERVERS

The number of persons observing each examination should be kept to a minimum. When observers are present, it is important to introduce these people to the patient. Only the person actually performing the test should communicate with the patient, as unnecessary talking can be disruptive and distressing. Questions or opinions voiced by observers can be misconstrued by the patient as an indication that he has some cardiac problem. All discussion should therefore be reserved until the examination is complete and the patient has left the area.

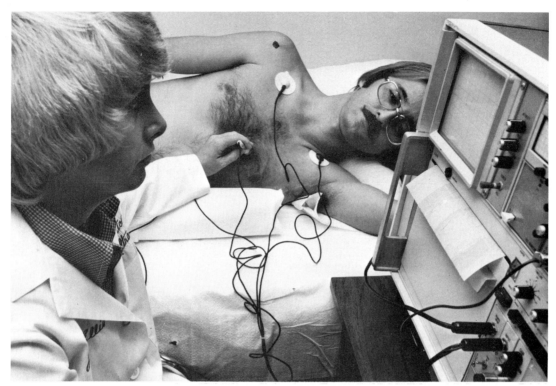

Figure 2–1.   The comfort of both the technologist and the patient is an important factor in producing an echocardiographic recording of good technical quality. The following features illustrate this. The patient is resting comfortably on his left side, thereby lessening the incidence of echocardiographic artifact due to muscle tension. The proximity of the technologist to both the patient and the ultrasound unit enables her to manage transducer placement with ease and, at the same time, to make the necessary control adjustments without disturbing the position of the transducer. The arm holding the transducer is resting on a rolled-up towel. In addition to relieving arm and shoulder tension, this also serves to stabilize management of the transducer.

The patient must never be placed in the position of feeling that he is a teaching object.

PATIENT DATA

Prior to the performance of an echocardiographic examination, the technologist should learn as much as possible about the patient. Knowledge of the reason the physician ordered the test allows the technologist to pay particular attention to the area of concern. For example, if the physician has noted a mid-systolic click, particular attention to the motion of the mitral leaflets during mid- and late systole may be critical.

In the case of the hospitalized patient, data can be obtained easily from the medical record. This will provide the technologist with a review of the patient's history and physical examination, the physician's progress notes, nurse's notes, and, in many cases, electrocardiographic and catheterization data. This information will usually provide an indication of what specific disorders the physician suspects if they are not stated on the echocardiogram order sheet. For example, it will be indicated if the patient has had a history of rheumatic fever, coronary disease, cardiac murmurs, or pericardial friction rub.

In the case of an out-patient for whom there is insufficient information on the prescription, the referring physician should be contacted. The technologist should learn what diagnoses the physician is considering. In the event that the physician cannot be consulted, tactful questioning of the patient may reveal why the test was ordered, but this approach should be a last resort.

In summary, the technologist should make every effort to see that the patient is relaxed and comfortable and to learn the pertinent facts of the patient's history before performing the echocardiographic test. These preliminaries greatly increase the chances of obtaining an adequate, informative scan.

TESTING ARRANGEMENT

Because of the duration of an echocardiographic examination (from 15 to 45 minutes), the comfort of both the technologist and the patient is important. Early fatigue on the part of the technologist is usually the result of discomfort and can result in a technically poor reading. To avoid this, the ultrasound unit should be positioned in such a way that the controls are within easy reach, so that adjustments can be made without changing the position of the transducer.

Arm and shoulder tension can be relieved by resting the arm used to hold the transducer on a rolled-up towel or a small pillow (see Figure 2–1). This is also more comfortable for the patient than having the examiner's arm resting on his chest. Whether the transducer is held in the right or the left hand or whether the patient is scanned from the right or the left side is a matter of individual technologist preference. For the purposes of this manual, however, the technologist will be shown positioned in a testing chair on the left side of the patient.

TRANSDUCER TECHNIQUE

Firm transducer placement is best maintained when the examiner places the base of his hand on the patient's chest and manipulates the probe with the thumb and first three fingers (Fig. 2–2). Because transmission gel is used, it is necessary to exert only enough pressure to maintain transducer control. After placing the transducer at the fourth intercostal space, 2 to 3 cm from the left sternal border, the transducer should not be "moved," but gently angled. This is especially important in scanning from one structure to another. Broad movements should be avoided, and only very slight, deliberate tilting motions should be made. Before changing slowly from one structure to another, it is important to note where and how the transducer is positioned. Then, if there is difficulty in locating the new struc-

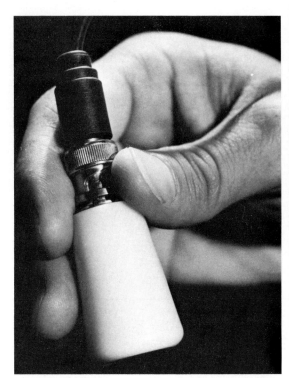

Figure 2–2.   The transducer is best controlled by holding it close to its base with the thumb and first three fingers. Using this technique, with the base of the hand resting on the patient's chest, the transducer may be manipulated easily.

ture, the transducer can be returned to its original position, and movement to the new structure can be repeated at a slightly different path of angulation.

TRANSDUCER PLACEMENT

Because the fourth intercostal space provides the largest "window," this is usually the best position from which to perform the examination. There are times, however, when the third or the fifth intercostal space will be used, even though these spaces usually provide considerably smaller windows. The other intercostal spaces on the left side are limited medially by the sternum, laterally and superiorly by the edge of the lung, and inferiorly by the boundary of the heart and diaphragm (Fig. 2–3).

The physical structure of the patient will suggest the best transducer placement. For example, in the obese person, the heart is usually horizontal, and the best initial trans-

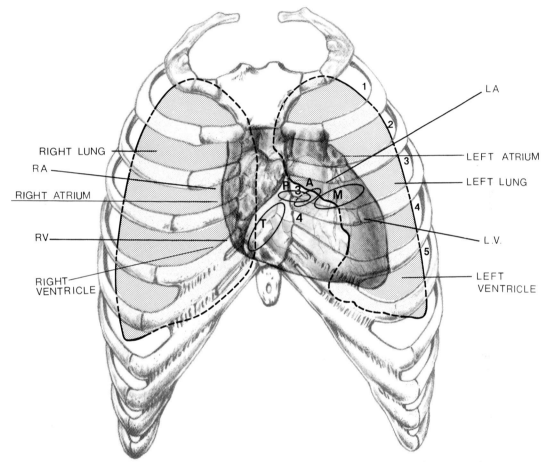

Figure 2–3. The fourth intercostal space (4) provides the largest cardiac "window." Because of the position of the lung (shaded area), the third (3) and fifth (5) intercostal spaces provide much smaller windows through which to perform the echocardiographic examination. In the chest cavity, note the approximate position of the heart chambers and valves in relation to the rib interspaces and lungs (T = tricuspid valve; P = pulmonary valve; A = aortic valve; M = mitral valve).

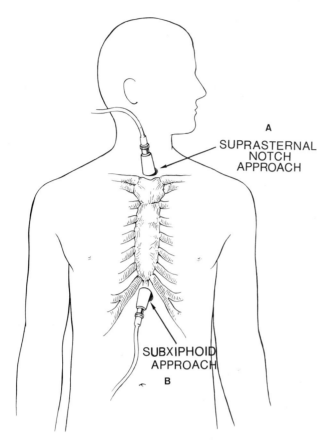

A
SUPRASTERNAL
NOTCH
APPROACH

SUBXIPHOID
APPROACH
B

Figure 2-4. Diagrammatic representation of correct transducer placement for (A) the suprasternal notch approach and (B) the subxiphoid approach.

ducer placement may be at the third intercostal space, 4 to 5 cm from the left sternal border. Tall, thin people tend to have vertical hearts, and a good starting position is often the fifth intercostal space, 1 to 2 cm from the left sternal border.

Patients with enlarged lungs caused by chronic obstructive lung disease present a unique problem. The multiple air-tissue interfaces in pulmonary tissue disperse the

ultrasound beam and prevent penetration. When the condition is severe, a low-frequency transducer (i.e., 1.6 MHz) should be used. If this approach is unsatisfactory, the examination should be performed from the subxiphoid position. This technique involves placing the transducer directly below the xiphoid process and aiming it upward toward the left shoulder in a "scooping" motion (Fig. 2–4). With this technique,

Figure 2–5. (A) When recorded from the subxiphoid position, the mitral valve (MV) will usually retain its normal echocardiographic "M"-shaped configuration. However, because the transducer is directed dramatically more superiorly and the ultrasound beam is not perpendicular to the structures involved, the mitral valve recording is not an optimal one, and the interventricular septum (IVS) is not clearly defined. (B) Subxiphoid recording of the aortic root. The echo-free space behind the posterior aortic root (PAR) is the main pulmonary artery (MPA), anterior to the wall of the left atrium (LAW). Using the subxiphoid position, the transducer is directed superiorly and passes through the right ventricle (RV), tricuspid valve (not seen), the aorta, and pulmonary artery (AAR = anterior aortic root). (C) The right and left ventricular chambers demonstrate a poorly defined interventricular septum (IVS), with no clear definition of the endocardial-epicardial echoes of the posterior left ventricular wall (PWLV). The combined obscureness of these necessary echoes prevents accurate measurement of both the right and left ventricular chambers (RVC = right ventricular chamber; LVC = left ventricular chamber).

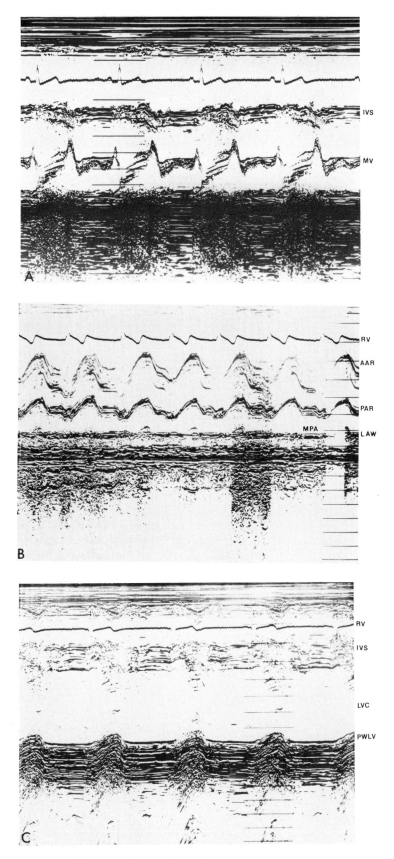

Figure 2–5. See legend on opposite page

13

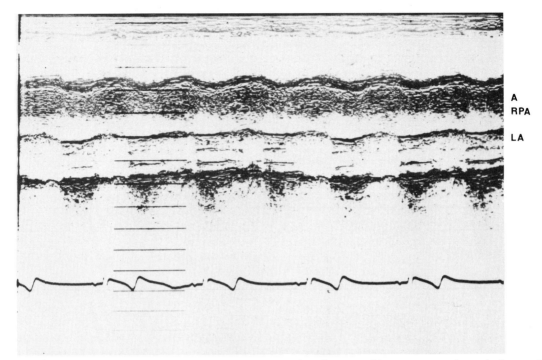

Figure 2–6. From the suprasternal notch position, the ultrasound beam passes through the aortic arch (A), the right pulmonary artery (RPA), and the left atrium (LA).

the transducer may have to be angled in many directions before a familiar pattern is recognized on the A-mode. Although it may not be possible to obtain accurate measurements of the right ventricle and left atrium, an otherwise valid examination can usually be performed from the subxiphoid position (Fig. 2–5).[1-3]

The suprasternal notch technique is another transducer placement variation that requires very careful angulation to avoid recording the trachea (see Figure 2–4). This involves gentle angulation of the transducer in an inferior direction and toward the heart. This technique is most useful in assessing a greatly enlarged left atrium, a condition that in some patients cannot be seen from the standard left parasternal approach. From the suprasternal notch, the transducer beam first strikes the aortic arch, then the right pulmonary artery, and finally, the left atrium (Fig. 2–6).[4] Because angulation of the transducer is rather limited in this area, the technique is difficult and should be employed only when the standard approach fails.

A STANDARDIZED ECHOCARDIOGRAM

There is no completely uniform approach to the performance of the echocardiographic examination. Patient positioning and instrumentation adjustment vary with each patient. The technologist must learn to recognize patterns of motion and to make adjustments accordingly. Refinement of this skill requires experience, good judgment, and patience.

Because all structures within the heart are functionally and anatomically interrelated, a complete echocardiographic examination should be routine. When there is one problem area, its effects will often be transmitted to other areas. For example, in severe mitral stenosis, the left atrium as well as the mitral valve will be affected. Recording only the mitral valve, therefore, would not reveal the extent of cardiac involvement. Furthermore, the presence of disease of other valves is often seen in association with mitral valve disease. Therefore, clear tracings of all valves should be attempted. A

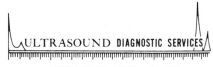

ULTRASOUND DIAGNOSTIC SERVICES

OSBORN MEDICAL CENTER   Suite 106
444 West Osborn Road
Phoenix, Arizona 85013
(602)   279-9375

DATE _____

CARDIAC ULTRASOUND REPORT

NAME _____ ECHO NO. _____ HEIGHT _____

DIAGNOSIS _____ WEIGHT _____

REASON FOR TEST _____ AGE _____

REFERRING PHYSICIAN _____ BSA _____ M²

Figure 2–7. Sample echo-cardiographic report form.

	MEASURED	(ADULT NORMAL)
MITRAL VALVE		
EF Slope (Diastolic Descent Rate)		(65-160 mm/sec)
Amplitude of Excursion		(17-25 mm)
AORTIC ROOT AND AORTIC VALVE		
End-Systolic Dimension		(2.7-3.6 cm)
Systolic Leaflet Separation		(1.7-2.2 cm)
LEFT ATRIUM		
Internal Dimension		(<4.0 cm)
Corrected for Body Surface Area		(<2.1 cm/M²)
LEFT VENTRICLE		
End-Diastolic Dimension		(<5.5 cm)
End-Systolic Dimension		(<4.0 cm)
Fractional Shortening		(>25%)
Ejection Time		
Mean Rate of Circum. Fiber Shortening (Vcf)		(0.9-1.8 cir/sec)
Septal Thickness		(<1.2 cm)
Posterior Wall Thickness		(<1.1 cm)
Septal: Posterior Wall Thickness (Ratio)		(<1.5:1)
RIGHT VENTRICLE		
Internal Dimension		(<3.0 cm)
Corrected for Body Surface Area		(<1.4 cm/M²)
PERICARDIAL EFFUSION		

IMPRESSION:

_____ , M.D.

routine complete echocardiographic examination includes recordings of the mitral valve, the aortic root, the aortic valve, the left atrium, the left ventricle, the interventricular septum, and the right ventricle. It is also advisable to attempt recordings of the tricuspid and pulmonic valves, although these are often more difficult to obtain, especially in adults.

It is helpful to have an echocardiographic form or worksheet at hand to note the de-tails of the examination. An example is included as Figure 2–7.

MEASUREMENTS

Understanding what data are required before valid measurements are made will enhance the technical quality of the recording. For this reason, the initial echocardiographic measurements should be made by the technologist.

To help insure accuracy in measuring, at least two recordings of each structure should be available for comparison. The mitral valve closing slope and amplitude can vary from recording to recording because of the dramatic range of motion of the valve leaflets. Motion, however, is not a factor in determining cardiac chamber size and wall thickness. Therefore, if two recordings of the same chamber have a variance of greater than 5 mm, a recording error, such as improper transducer angulation, or a measuring error, such as misidentification of the endocardial edge of the chamber, has probably occurred. The physician interpreting the examination can remeasure questionable and important portions of the recording. Ideally, this should be done in the presence of the technologist, who can clarify such technical aspects of the examination as patient position, problems encountered, and transducer technique. This type of interchange between the physician and the technologist is necessary to derive optimal data from the echocardiogram.

INSTRUMENTATION

Because control settings differ from patient to patient, they should not be preset. It is also imperative that the technologist have a good working knowledge as to what the controls do, especially since the proper adjustment for each individual patient is crucial for proper technique. Although the use of these controls is repeatedly illustrated in subsequent chapters, their function will be more clearly discussed under this section on instrumentation (Fig. 2–8).

The Echocardiographic Controls

MODES. The typical pulse-echo system utilizes two types of output display. The first of these, the A-mode display, is seen on the oscilloscope as a series of vertical sig-

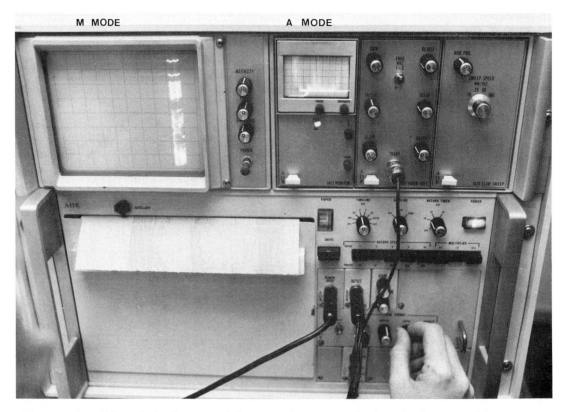

Figure 2–8. Although the location of the controls varies with ultrasound unit models, the instrumentation shown gives an example of the controls found on the majority of ultrasound units. Note the presence of both the M-mode and the A-mode displays.

nals rising immediately above the base line (see Figure 1–3). The stronger echoes are represented by taller spikes, the less intense by shorter spikes. The spikes move in rhythm with the heart and have definite pattern configurations that correspond to the various cardiac structures. Therefore, it is good practice to preview in A-mode for positive identification of the structure to be recorded before observation of the M-mode presentation.

The second and most commonly used display for cardiac evaluation is the M-mode or time-motion (T-M) display. This type of display is usually presented on the cathode-ray tube as the motion of the echoes is tracked and recorded on a strip-chart recorder to produce a time-motion wave form. Because of the dynamic motion of the heart, the analysis of its component structures as they move in time provides an essential dimension in cardiac ultrasonic evaluation.

INTENSITY. Determines the brightness of the trace.

SWEEP SPEED. Establishes the rate (mm/sec) at which the trace sweeps repetitively.

PAPER SPEED. A prerequisite of an echocardiographic recorder is availability of variable paper speeds. Some techniques require a recording speed as slow as 10 mm/sec, while others may require a speed of 100 mm/sec or more. Thus, a satisfactory strip-chart recorder should have the ability to vary the paper speed fairly widely. A convenience that facilitates the interpretation of many echocardiograms is vertical time lines. This feature enhances the ability to correlate the timing of electrocardiographic and echocardiographic events.

REJECT. The reject control is employed to eliminate low-amplitude signals. Optimally, it is used to produce a more refined, less cluttered recording, which is particularly helpful in eliminating unimportant intracavitary echoes (presumably from blood or lung interference). Caution should always be exercised when using reject, in view of the fact that too much reject can eliminate the relatively weak echoes, such as those reflected from the endocardium. Furthermore, abnormally thickened structures, such as a fibrosed, stenotic mitral valve, can be made to appear as very thin echoes (see Figure 4–49).

GAIN. Without changing the intensity of the sound energy produced, the gain control permits an increase in the electronic signal strength of the received echoes. Some manufacturers use the term "attenuation" for the same function.

There are usually two types of gain incorporated into every cardiac ultrasound system — near and overall gain. The overall gain permits a uniform increase in the size of all signals. Thus, higher gains are required for thick chest walls and weakly reflecting structures such as the aortic valve. Conversely, lower gains, by decreasing the amplitude of the echoes, will minimize the display of weak, cluttering echo signals that arise from multiple reflections within tissue such as chest and heart walls.

The overall gain alone, however, does not provide adequate adjustment of signal level for display of structures in the near ranges. If overall gain were the only gain available, the echoes in the near ranges would appear extremely large, and the far echoes would be small. More specifically, the structures near the chest wall would be very intense in relation to those from more distant structures of similar density. To overcome this problem, a compensation technique is used that permits gain to be increased for signals more distant from the transducer. This compensation circuit is commonly referred to as "time gain compensation" (TGC), "depth compensation," or "distance compensation."

A near-field gain control (the delay) reduces the large signals and enables the technologist to compensate for this effect by specifying the degree of suppression as well as the range over which it is effective. The range over which the gain of the far echoes is increased is varied by the slope. The greatest artifactual error induced by incorrect use of this control is the elimination of a portion of the echoes from the interventricular septum (see Figure 8–16).

DAMPING. This control is not available on all cardiac ultrasound systems. Electronically, it reduces the sound energy output by decreasing the input pulse width to the transducer. This control provides an excellent means for proper structure identification. For example, the strong pericardial echo can be isolated from the posterior wall of the left ventricle, and the thickness of the pericardium can be assessed.

DELAY. On some cardiac ultrasound systems, the delay is referred to as the *start*. On systems used exclusively for echocardiography, this control requires little or no adjustment and sets the oscilloscope position of the "main bang," the echo representation of the skin-transducer interface.

DEPTH. This setting should be adjusted to where the entire heart is seen on the scope. The total depth of field may be increased or decreased by this control. For example, by extreme scale expansion, the entire field could be set to look only at the aortic root, with no visualization of the left atrial wall. Conversely, adjusting this control to a point where the heart structures are compressed too closely together will result in poor visualization and resolution.

ELECTROCARDIOGRAM GAIN AND POSITION. Every echocardiogram should include a simultaneous recording of an electrocardiographic lead. The simultaneous electrocardiogram demonstrates alterations

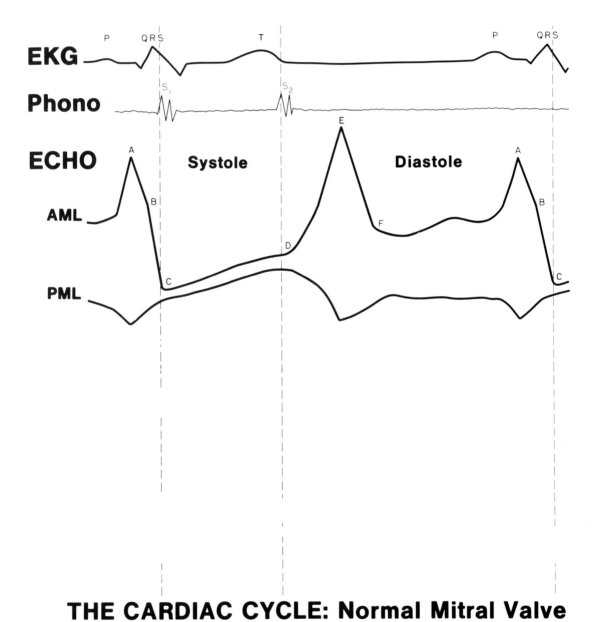

THE CARDIAC CYCLE: Normal Mitral Valve

Figure 2-9. Schematic representation demonstrating the correct location of the electrocardiogram and phonocardiogram in relation to the echocardiogram.

in valve and wall motion caused by arrhythmias and permits timing of cardiac anatomical events in terms of the electrical activity of the heart (see Chapter 3, "The Electrocardiogram and the Echocardiogram"). Ideally, the electrocardiogram should be positioned in a clear space immediately above the echocardiographic trace. Furthermore, the gain should be adjusted so that the QRS complex of the electrocardiogram is large enough to be easily seen. In the event that the ultrasound system has phonocardiogram capabilities, the phono trace should be positioned immediately below the electro-cardiogram, also in an echo-free space (Fig. 2–9).

REFERENCES

1. Chang S, and Feigenbaum H: Subxiphoid echocardiography. J Clin Ultrasound 1:14–20, 1973.
2. Chang S, Feigenbaum H, and Dillon JC: Subxiphoid echocardiography: A review. Chest 68:233, 1975.
3. Feigenbaum H: Echocardiography. Philadelphia, Lea and Febiger, 1976.
4. Goldberg BB: Suprasternal ultrasonography. JAMA 215:245–250, 1971.

Chapter 3

THE ELECTROCARDIOGRAM AND THE ECHOCARDIOGRAM

The diagnostic value of echocardiography relies not only upon the precise application of ultrasound technology but also upon careful interpretation of test results in light of other means of cardiac evaluation. No test is more important in the correct interpretation of the echocardiogram than the electrocardiogram. In many instances, echocardiographic findings gain added meaning when a full, 12-lead, scalar electrocardiogram is available to demonstrate patterns such as infarction, bundle branch block, and muscular hypertrophy. Furthermore, the echocardiogram must always include simultaneous recording of a single electrocardiographic lead, preferably lead II.

The simultaneous one-lead recording will reveal any disturbances in heart rhythm that occur during the course of the echocardiographic examination. Such changes can have a profound effect on the motion of the walls and valves of the heart. Thus, consequent echocardiographic aberrations must be interpreted in light of associated electrocardiographic changes (Fig. 3–1). In addition, the ECG provides an important reference point for those measurements requiring the timing of cardiac events.

The electrocardiographic recording should be positioned so that the echoes originating from the cardiac structures are not obscured. With the newer recorders, it can be placed entirely outside the echocardiogram. When this is not possible, the electrocardiogram should be positioned within the echo-free right ventricular or left ventricular chamber.

THE NORMAL MITRAL VALVE

Of the cardiac structures that are routinely recorded, the normal mitral valve has the greatest range of motion throughout the cardiac cycle. For that reason, it provides the best example of the relationship between the events of the electrocardiogram and the echocardiogram. This relationship is depicted in Figure 3–2.

The Normal Mitral Valve in Cardiac Arrhythmias

In cases of sinus tachycardia, atrial fibrillation, and atrial flutter, when the ventricular rate is sufficiently rapid, the mitral valve may exhibit only a single opening during ventricular diastole.[1, 2] A single diastolic opening motion may also be seen in atrioventricular heart block and both premature atrial and ventricular contractions.[3] Examples illustrating the effects of arrhythmias on the motion of the mitral valve are provided in Figures 3–3 to 3–7.

THE AORTIC ROOT AND VALVE

The motion of the aortic root is the same as that of the cardiac skeleton — anterior in direction during ventricular systole and posterior in direction during early diastole.[4] On the optimal aortic root recording, at least some portion of the aortic valve leaflets is apparent, the walls are thin and distinct,

Text continued on page 28

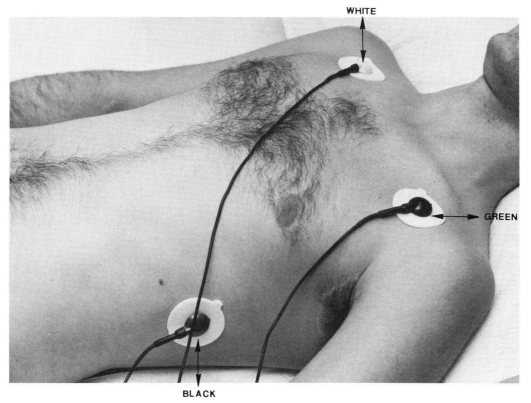

Figure 3-1. To obtain the simultaneous electrocardiogram, the technologist can best rely on the color-coded leads. A simulated lead-II recording may be made by placing the green electrode at the region of the mid-clavicular line, the white electrode at the right mid-clavicular line, and the black electrode along the left lateral side. This electrode placement also aids in reducing electrocardiogram artifact from muscle tension.

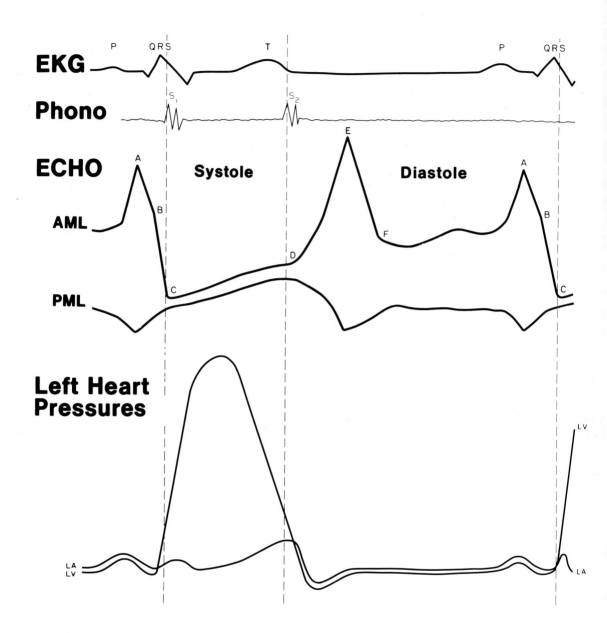

THE CARDIAC CYCLE: Normal Mitral Valve

Figure 3–2.   The echocardiographic A wave following the P wave of the electrocardiogram occurs during atrial contraction. C represents mitral valve closure occurring during the electrocardiographic QRS complex. D-E represents rapid valve opening following the T wave of the electrocardiogram in diastole. E-F (diastole) represents semi-closure of the mitral valve immediately after rapid ventricular filling.

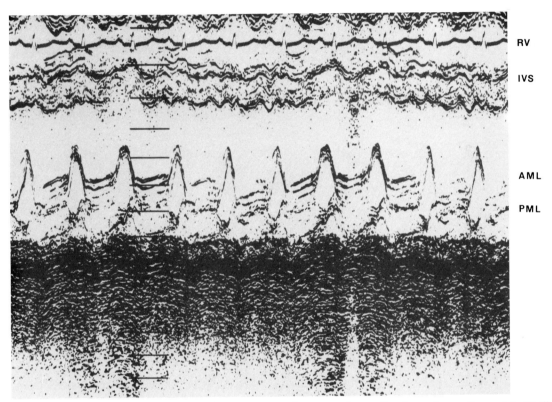

RV

IVS

AML

PML

Figure 3–3. Sinus tachycardia. In the presence of sinus tachycardia, the echocardiographic "M" configuration of the mitral valve is lost as ventricular diastole is dramatically shortened. Furthermore, the mitral F point is lost as the E and A waves merge (RV = right ventricle; IVS = interventricular septum; AML = anterior mitral leaflet; PML = posterior mitral leaflet).

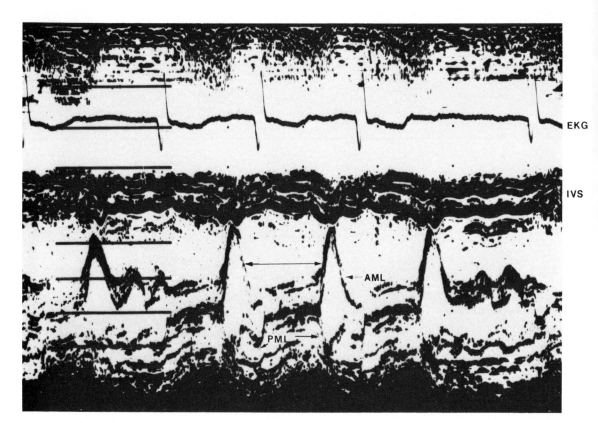

Figure 3–4. In atrial fibrillation, a true A wave is absent. Short opening motions are often seen during long diastolic periods, but may be missing when the electrocardiographic (EKG) R-R intervals are shortened, as depicted in the 2nd and 3rd mitral valve complexes (arrow). Note the normal double opening of the posterior mitral leaflets (PML) even when the anterior leaflet (AML) shows only a single opening (IVS = interventricular septum).

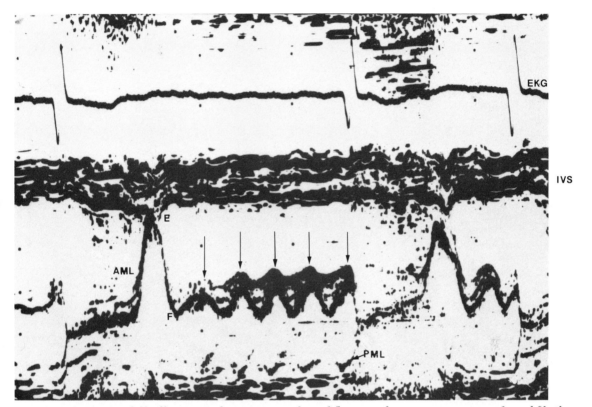

Figure 3–5. Atrial fibrillation. In the presence of atrial flutter and, in many instances of atrial fibrillation, the echocardiographic appearance of the normal mitral valve is characterized by pronounced coarse oscillations (arrows) during long R-R diastolic intervals. The mitral valve remains partially closed during this fluttering and closes completely with the onset of ventricular systole (QRS complex of the electrocardiogram) (IVS = interventricular septum; AML = anterior mitral leaflet; PML = posterior mitral leaflet).

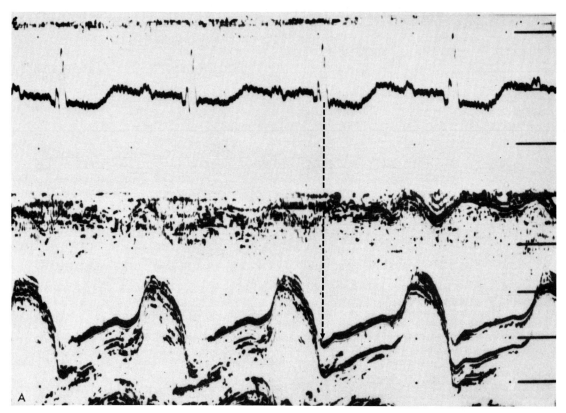

Figure 3–6. (A) In first degree heart block (prolonged P-R interval), atrial contraction occurs early, causing the two phases of ventricular filling to merge, and the distinct mitral A wave is lost (arrow). In this recording, the P-R interval is only slightly prolonged. Although mitral valve closure occurs normally at the onset of the QRS complex (dotted line), the E and A waves merge, resulting in a single diastolic opening.

Illustration continued on opposite page

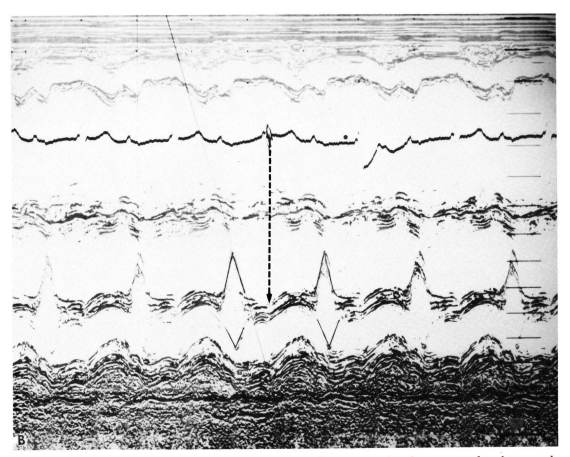

Figure 3–6 Continued. (B) A more severely prolonged P-R interval is demonstrated in this recording. Mitral valve closure clearly precedes the electrocardiographic QRS complex (dotted line). The electrocardiogram is essential in the presence of the single-opening mitral valve because it documents the early contraction that results from first-degree block.

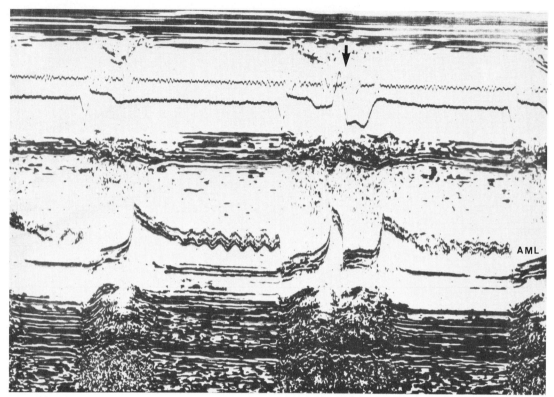

AML

Figure 3–7. A premature ventricular beat in atrial fibrillation. Multiple oscillations of the anterior mitral leaflet (AML) are seen during diastole. No distinct A wave is seen. A premature ventricular contraction (arrow) causes early closure after the second beat.

and all portions of the normal wall motion are visualized.

The dimension of the aortic root varies with the cardiac cycle. The largest dimension occurs at the time of maximal anterior displacement, immediately following ventricular ejection (following the T wave of the electrocardiogram).

The narrowest dimension occurs immediately preceding ventricular systole, at the commencement of the electrocardiographic QRS complex. The latter is the single most reproducible echocardiographic measurement, because it is the least affected by stroke volume and cardiac rotation, and it is taken at a fixed point in the cardiac cycle with reference to the electrocardiogram (Fig. 3–8).

In diastole, between the electrocardiographic T wave and the beginning of the QRS complex, the aortic valve leaflets are in the closed position, forming a roughly single plane parallel to the ultrasound beam. The result is a thin band of echoes in approximately the center of the aortic root, moving parallel with the aortic root walls. With the onset of left ventricular systole, the three leaflets diverge onto three separate planes as the valve opens. In their open position, the posterior (noncoronary) cusp lies adjacent to the posterior aortic wall, the right cusp is next to the anterior wall, and the left cusp echo appears between the posterior and right cusps. The resultant configuration is a box-like appearance of the aortic cusp motion in ventricular systole (Fig. 3–8). In this open phase, the separation between the right coronary and the posterior cusps remains constant, or narrows slightly during systole, and normally ranges from 1.7 to 2.5 cm.

As demonstrated in Figures 3–9 to 3–12, the effects of arrhythmias are also visible on the recordings of the aortic root and aortic valve.[5, 6]

THE LEFT ATRIUM

Echocardiographically, the anterior left atrial wall is inseparable from the posterior wall of the aortic root. A distinctive, three-

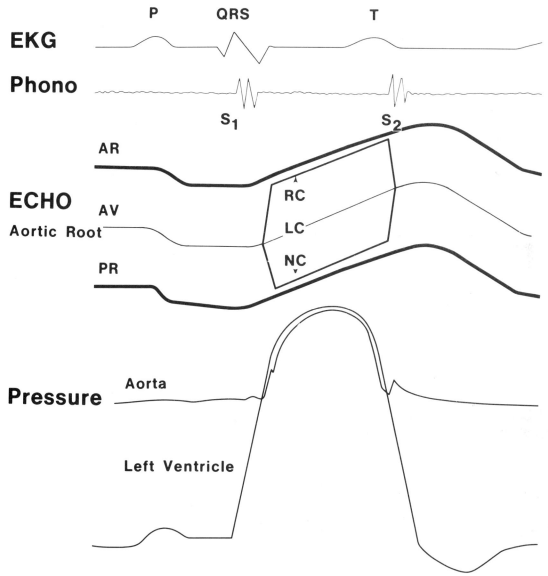

Figure 3–8. The motion of the aortic root and aortic valve during the cardiac cycle. At the end of systole, the aortic root reaches its peak anterior displacement and also attains its largest dimension. At end-diastole, at the commencement of the electrocardiographic QRS complex, the aortic root reaches its narrowest dimension. The aortic valve (AV) opens following the electrocardiographic QRS complex (systole). From top to bottom, the right coronary (RC), the left coronary (LC), and the non-coronary (NC) cusps are seen in their fully open positions during ventricular systole. Note that all three leaflets merge approximately in the center of the aorta during diastole. Also during diastole, the motion of the closed leaflets parallels that of the aortic walls.

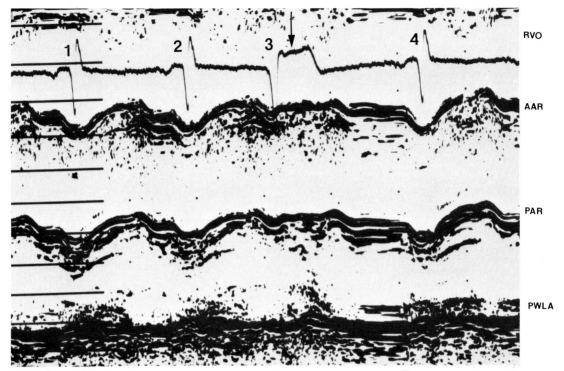

Figure 3-9. The effect of a premature beat on the motion of the normal aortic root. Prior to the second beat (2), the anterior (AAR) and posterior (PAR) walls of the aortic root move in a normal parallel fashion. However, as a result of a premature beat (3), the walls of the aortic root exhibit a prolonged blunted appearance. With contraction of the fourth beat (4), normal motion is resumed (PWLA = posterior wall of left atrium; RVO = right ventricular outflow tract).

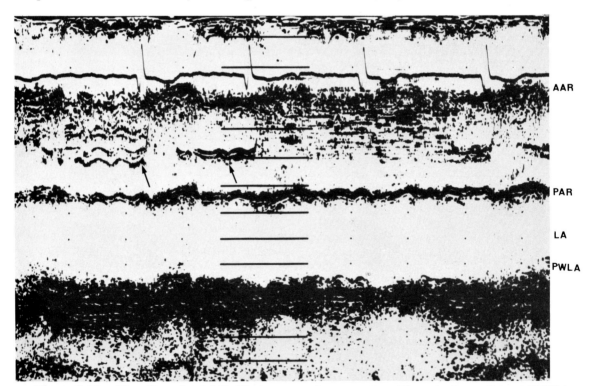

Figure 3-10. The effect of atrial fibrillation on aortic root motion. The anterior aortic root (AAR) is partially obscured. The posterior aortic root (PAR) appears as an undulating line, being most pronounced during diastole (arrows). These diastolic undulations are also reflected during the closing phase of the aortic valve (arrows) (LA = left atrium; PWLA = posterior wall of the left atrium).

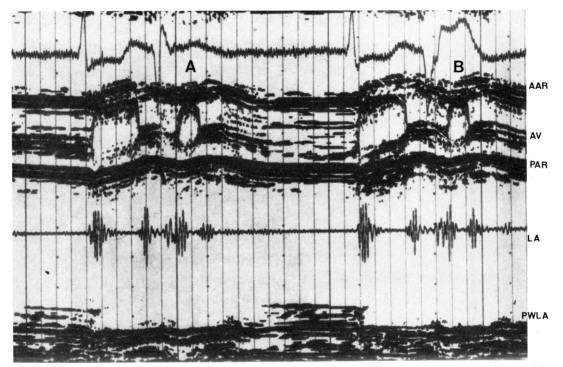

Figure 3-11. The aortic valve with premature beats. The normal cardiac cycle is interrupted by premature contractions (A and B). While the first and third beats exhibit normal opening, the second and fourth beats (A and B) are associated with a shortened duration of valve opening (AAR = anterior aortic root wall; AV = aortic valve; PAR = posterior aortic root wall; LA = left atrium; PWLA = posterior wall of the left atrium).

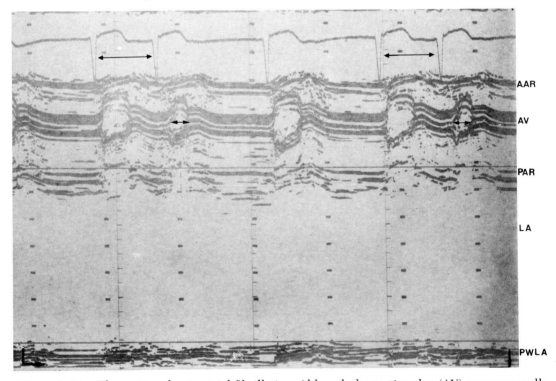

Figure 3-12. The aortic valve in atrial fibrillation. Although the aortic valve (AV) opens normally with the QRS complex and closes following the electrocardiographic T wave, the duration of its opening is proportional to the duration of each previous R-R interval (arrows). The left atrium is severely dilated (AAR = anterior aortic root wall; PAR = posterior aortic root wall; PWLA = posterior wall of the left atrium).

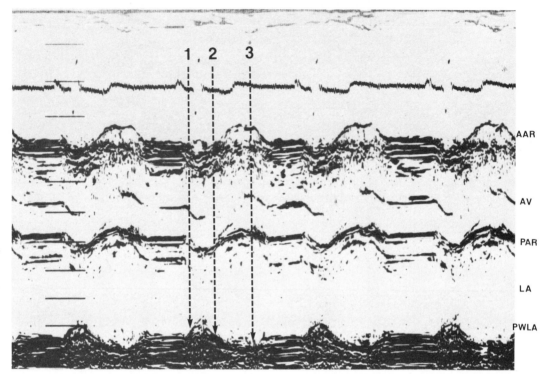

Figure 3–13.   The motion of the left atrial wall (PWLA) in relation to the electrocardiogram. The three segments representing the motion of the left atrial wall include (arrows) (1) anterior motion following the electrocardiographic P wave; (2) posterior motion following the QRS complex of the electrocardiogram; (3) following the posterior motion, a period of short, abrupt anterior motion (AAR = anterior aortic root; AV = aortic valve; PAR = posterior aortic root wall; LA = left atrium; PWLA = posterior wall of the left atrium).

phase motion pattern indicative of volume changes within the left atrial chamber often becomes apparent when recorded near the mitral orifice:

1. Anterior motion following the onset of the electrocardiographic P wave (the left atrium begins contracting after the right atrium). This contraction of the left atrial wall may appear rounded or may exhibit a sharp, peaked appearance on the echocardiogram. The motion occurs slightly after the mitral A wave.

2. Posterior motion following the QRS complex of the electrocardiogram during ventricular systole as the left atrium fills with blood returning from the lungs. A bulging of the mitral leaflets as a result of high left ventricular pressure effectively reduces left atrial chamber size, and this also probably contributes to the posterior excursion of the left atrial wall.

3. A short, abrupt anterior displacement

after mitral valve opening as blood enters the ventricle from the atrium.

The relationship of the electrocardiogram to these three phases is illustrated in Figure 3–13.

THE INTERVENTRICULAR SEPTUM

When the transducer is directed through the midportion of the left ventricle, the interventricular septum appears as two parallel lines moving anteriorly during ventricular diastole, just after the electrocardiographic inscription of the P wave. This anterior motion continues for 0.04 to 0.06 second after the onset of the QRS complex of the electrocardiogram. The septum then moves posteriorly and thickens during ventricular systole (Fig. 3–14), followed by a relatively flat motion, except for a small

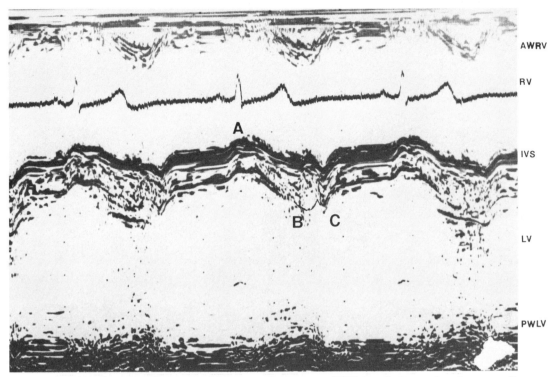

AWRV

RV

IVS

LV

PWLV

Figure 3–14.   The normal motion of the muscular septum (IVS) in relation to the electrocardiogram. (A) Following the inscription of the P wave of the electrocardiogram, the septum moves abruptly anteriorly until after the onset of the QRS complex. (B) After the onset of the QRS complex, the septum moves posteriorly and thickens until just after the T wave of the electrocardiogram. (C) Septal relaxation, which is sometimes interrupted by a small notch (AWRV = anterior wall of right ventricle; PWLV = posterior wall of the left ventricle).

early diastolic notch, during diastole prior to atrial contraction.[7]

THE POSTERIOR LEFT VENTRICULAR WALL

Posterior left ventricular wall motion occurs in three phases coincident with ventricular systole, early diastole, and mid-late diastole.[8]

1. Ventricular systole. The posterior wall of the left ventricle moves anteriorly as a result of myocardial fiber shortening and consequent wall thickening. The anterior displacement is also partially due to the motion of the entire heart during ventricular systole. At the peak of its anterior excursion, the aortic valve closes, and a short, slow posterior motion (isovolumetric relaxation) begins diastole.

2. Early diastole. The mitral valve opens, and the posterior wall of the left ventricle

quickly moves posteriorly during the period of rapid ventricular filling.

3. Mid-late diastole. The posterior wall of the left ventricle moves slowly posteriorly following the period of rapid filling for the duration of diastole (Fig. 3–15).

EFFECTS OF ARRHYTHMIAS ON THE INTERVENTRICULAR SEPTUM AND POSTERIOR LEFT VENTRICULAR WALL

As discussed earlier in this chapter, cardiac rhythm, particularly marked alterations in the length of the R-R interval, and the type of arterial activity and synchronization of atrial and ventricular contractions affect the motion of the cardiac valves. The effects of the cardiac rhythm on the echocardiographic pattern of the interventricular septum and the posterior left ventricular wall must also be recognized. Examples of the

Text continued on page 38

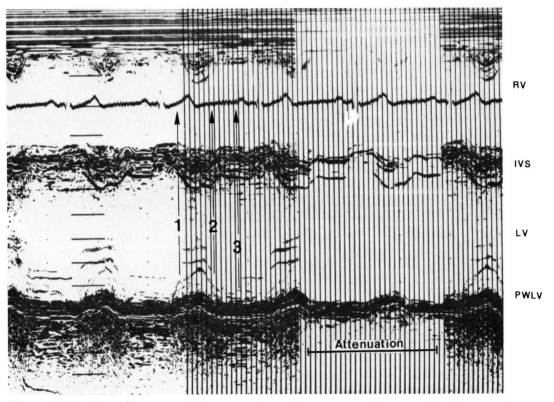

Figure 3-15.   Normal posterior left ventricular wall motion in relation to the electrocardiogram may be divided into three phases (arrows): (1) Ventricular systole: The start of anterior motion toward the septum (IVS). (2) Early diastole: Rapid motion posteriorly. (3) Mid-late diastole: Slow motion posteriorly for the duration of diastole (RV = right ventricle; LV = left ventricle; PWLV = posterior wall of the left ventricle).

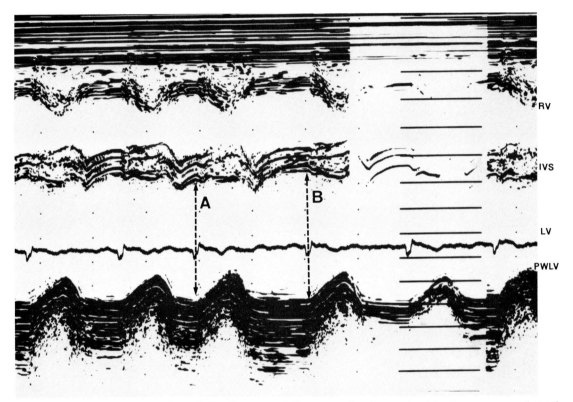

Figure 3–16. The effect of atrial fibrillation on left ventricular dimension.[8] In the presence of atrial fibrillation, there is a varying diastolic filling time of the left ventricle. Following a short R-R interval, the end-diastolic dimension is approximately 4.4 cm (A). After the longer cycle that follows, however, this dimension (B) has increased to approximately 5.0 cm as a result of a longer period of ventricular filling. There is abnormal, flattened septal motion due to coronary artery disease (RV = right ventricle; IVS = interventricular septum; LV = left ventricle; PWLV = posterior wall of the left ventricle).

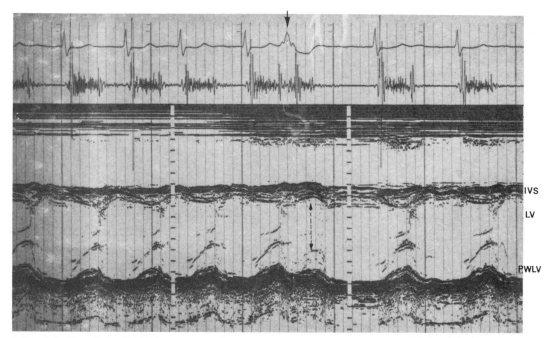

Figure 3–17. Septal (IVS) motion in the presence of a premature contraction. The interruption of a premature beat (arrow) causes the septum to move abruptly anteriorly, paralleling the motion of the posterior left ventricular wall (PWLV) (dotted line).

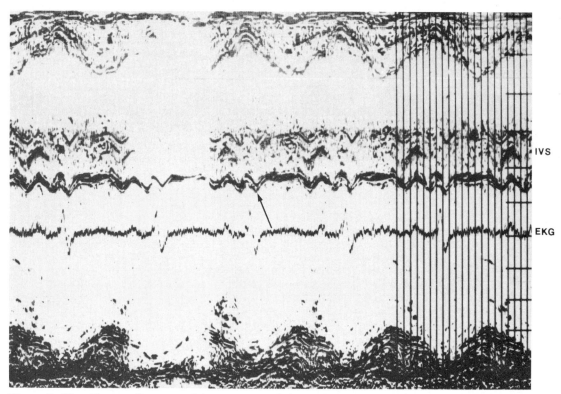

Figure 3–18. Abnormal motion of the septum in left bundle branch block.[9, 10, 11] Normally, contraction of the myocardial elements of the septum is preceded by electrical depolarization, which progresses from left to right. Alteration of electrical conduction, as in left bundle branch block, causes changes in the timing of septal contraction. In this recording, the septum typically exhibits a marked posterior displacement approximately 0.04 second after the onset of the QRS complex of the electrocardiogram (EKG) (arrow), corresponding to the pre-ejection period of left ventricular systole. Immediately following this abnormal posterior displacement (arrow), the septum (IVS) exhibits a flattened motion during the period of left ventricular ejection.

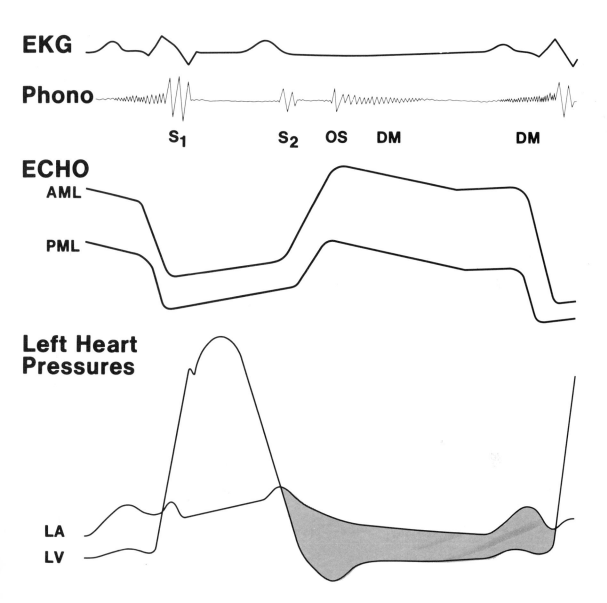

EKG

Phono

S₁ S₂ OS DM DM

ECHO

AML

PML

Left Heart Pressures

LA
LV

THE CARDIAC CYCLE: Mitral Stenosis

Figure 3–19. Schematic representation of mitral stenosis. Compared to the normal mitral valve (Fig. 3–2), pressure equalization between the atrium and ventricle does not occur when the valve opens (shaded area), resulting in a continuous blood flow across a pressure gradient, which, in severe stenosis, persists throughout diastole. The opening snap (OS) is related to the end of the rapid opening movement of the valve.

effects of various arrhythmias on these structures are presented in Figures 3–16 to 3–18.[9-11]

PHONOCARDIOGRAM, ELECTROCARDIOGRAM, AND ECHOCARDIOGRAM

Phonocardiography is the technique by which the sounds originating from the heart and great vessels are amplified and recorded on paper in a graphic representation. The added information of recording a simultaneous phonocardiogram with a lead-II electrocardiogram and echocardiogram is useful in many instances in the timing of heart sounds and murmurs (see Figure 3–2).[12, 13]

Recording Sites for Accurate Identification of Heart Sounds

Optimal transducer placement for recording heart sounds and murmurs often requires assistance from the physician. An example of the value of a simultaneous phonocardiogram is recording the opening snap of mitral stenosis (Fig. 3–19). Placement of the phonocardiographic transducer at the apex of the heart will usually provide maximum identificaton of the opening snap and murmur, and in most cases, this is best brought out by having the patient lie on his left side. This same position, at the apex, is also the best placement for the phonocardiographic transducer in recording mitral insufficiency, in which the murmur is caused by a reflux of blood through the mitral valve during systole.

Sounds originating from the left ventricular outflow tract, which includes the aortic valve, are best recorded high along the left sternal border and in the second right intercostal space. Tricuspid and right ventricular sounds are generally best detected low along the left sternal border.

REFERENCES

1. Edler I, Gustafson A, Karlefors T, and Christensson B: Ultrasoundcardiography. Acta Med Scand 170(Suppl 370):1, 1961.
2. Gabor GE, and Winsberg F: Motion of mitral valves in cardiac arrythmias (sic): Ultrasonic cardiographic study. Invest Radiol 5:355–360, 1970.
3. Shah PM, Kramer DH, and Gramiak R: Influence of the timing of atrial systole on mitral valve closure and on the first heart sound in man. Am J Cardiol 26:231, 1970.
4. Gramiak R, and Shah PM: Echocardiography of the aortic root. Invest Radiol 3:356–366, 1968.
5. Anastassiades PC, Quinones MA, Gaasch WH, et al.: Relation of aortic valve closure to the second heart sound: Echocardiographic and phonocardiographic assessment (Abstr). Circulation (Suppl III) 49,50:85, 1974.
6. Paraskos JA, and Montesclaros LA: Relation of the second heart sound to aortic valve closure as assessed by echocardiography (Abstr). Circulation (Suppl III) 49,50:239, 1974.
7. McDonald IG, Feigenbaum H, and Chang S: Analysis of the left ventricular wall motion by reflected ultrasound: Application to assessment of myocardial function. Circulation 46:14–25, 1972.
8. Redwood DR, Henry WL, and Epstein SE: Evaluation of the ability of echocardiography to measure acute alterations in left ventricular volume. Circulation 50:901–904, 1974.
9. Abbasi AS, Eber LM, MacAlpin RN, and Kattus AA: Paradoxical motion of interventricular septum in left bundle branch block. Circulation 49:423–427, 1974.
10. McDonald IG: Echocardiographic demonstration of abnormal motion of the interventricular septum in left bundle branch block. Circulation 48:272–280, 1972.
11. Dillon JC, Chang S, and Feigenbaum H: Echocardiographic manifestations of left bundle branch block. Circulation 49:876–880, 1974.
12. Waider W, and Craige E: First heart sound and ejection sounds: Echocardiographic and phonocardiographic correlation with valvular events. Am J Cardiol 35:346–356, 1975.
13. Burggraf GW, and Craige E: The first heart sound in complete heart block. Circulation 50:17–24, 1974.

Chapter 4

THE MITRAL VALVE

Through the pioneering work of Edler and Hertz,[1] the mitral valve was the first structure to receive detailed study by echocardiography, and much was learned about its physiology and pathophysiology. Its strategic position within the left side of the heart makes it the most important intracardiac structure to be studied by cardiac ultrasound. Not only does its motion reflect the function of the valve itself, but it also reflects the hemodynamics of the left atrium and left ventricle. For these reasons, it is fortunate that the mitral valve is one of the easiest of the cardiac structures to record.

ANATOMY

The mitral valve is the passageway through which blood is transported from the left atrium into the left ventricle. The anatomical structure of this valve allows it to prevent a back-flow of blood into the left atrium. It is composed primarily of two major leaflets, one anterior and one posterior, with the anterior leaflet being much longer from base to apex. These leaflets are interconnected by structures known as the commissures (designated anterolateral and posteromedial) and by the commissural leaflets.

The anterior mitral leaflet hangs like a curtain between the mitral and aortic orifices and is partially attached to the anterolateral wall of the left ventricle. This leaflet is continuous with the supporting tissues of the noncoronary and left coronary cusps of the aortic valve. The shorter posterior mitral leaflet originates from the lateral portion of the mitral ring and has less excursion than the anterior leaflet. In systole, when the valve closes, the larger anterior leaflet

"molds" to meet the smaller posterior leaflet. When this occurs and is viewed from the left atrium, the mitral valve takes on a crescent-shaped appearance (Fig. 4–1).

The mitral leaflets are connected to the papillary muscles in the left ventricular wall by strong fibrous cords called the chordae tendineae. Because they are located on the inner wall of the ventricle, they serve as "guy wires," tightening as the papillary muscles begin their contraction early in ventricular systole and thus helping to hold the cusps together and preventing eversion of the leaflets into the left atrium as the pressure rises in the ventricle. As the left ventricle contracts, so do the papillary muscles, thereby increasing the restraining action of the chordae tendineae, so that the upward merging of the leaflets occludes the mitral orifice.

In summary, there are four necessary factors involved in the function of the normal mitral valve: (1) there must be adequate pliability and disposition of the valve leaflets in relation to each other; (2) the chordae tendineae must be of proper length and originate from their corresponding papillary muscle; (3) the papillary muscles must contract and be appropriately situated in the left ventricular wall; and (4) in order for the cusps to meet, the mitral annulus must maintain its proper size (Fig. 4–2).

ECHOCARDIOGRAPHIC APPEARANCE

A-Mode Appearance

The mitral valve is recognized as the cardiac structure with the greatest amplitude of movement. In contrast to the subtle motion

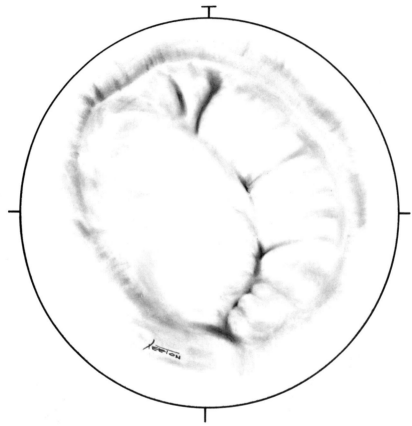

Figure 4-1.   Illustration of the mitral leaflets during closure. Viewed through the left atrium, the mitral valve appears as a crescent-shaped structure as the leaflets "mold" together to form a perfect seal at the time of closure.

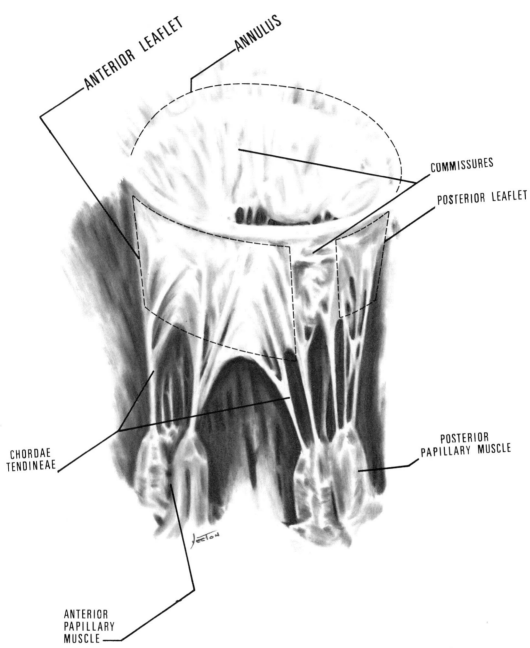

ANTERIOR LEAFLET

ANNULUS

COMMISSURES

POSTERIOR LEAFLET

CHORDAE
TENDINEAE

POSTERIOR
PAPILLARY MUSCLE

ANTERIOR
PAPILLARY
MUSCLE

Figure 4–2. Illustration of the mitral apparatus viewed from the posterolateral projection. Depicted are the anatomical components necessary for normal mitral function. Note the funnel-shaped appearance of the mitral valve in its opened position.

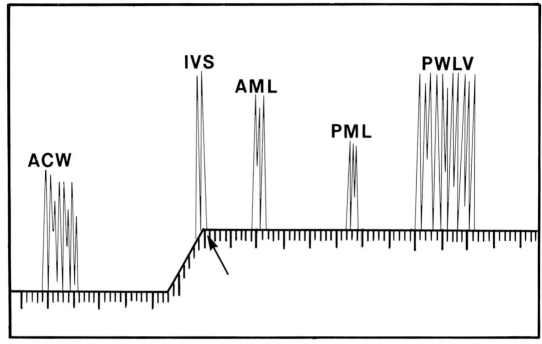

Figure 4–3. A-mode representation of the anterior and posterior leaflets of the mitral valve. Key: ACW = anterior chest wall; IVS = interventricular septum; AML = anterior mitral leaflet; PML = posterior mitral leaflet; PWLV = posterior wall of the left ventricle. Note the position of the TGC curve resting against the leading edge of the interventricular septum (arrow).

of the aortic root and the interventricular septum, the mitral valve has a far greater range of anterior-posterior motion. On the A-mode display, the tall, rapidly moving spike representing the anterior leaflet of the mitral valve can be seen exhibiting a "whip-like" motion between the interventricular septum and the posterior wall of the left ventricle. Motion toward the interventricular septum, or anteriorly, represents the opening of the valve. Conversely, motion posteriorly, or toward the left ventricular wall, represents closure of the valve.

The posterior mitral leaflet is seen between the anterior mitral leaflet and the posterior wall of the left ventricle, moving opposite to the anterior leaflet, although with considerably less amplitude (Fig. 4–3).

M-Mode Appearance

The anterior mitral leaflet on the M-mode display can best be described as a double peaked structure that roughly resembles a capital "M." This distinctive appearance can be found consistently in echocardiographic recordings of normal individuals.

Before describing the motion of the anterior leaflet in detail, it will be helpful to describe its related structures, including the interventricular septum, the right ventricle, the left ventricle, and the left atrium.

As shown in Figure 4–4, the structure closest to the anterior mitral leaflet during diastole is the interventricular septum. This is recognized as two more or less parallel echoes moving just anterior to the anterior mitral leaflet. As discussed in Chapter 8 ("The Interventricular Septum"), the septum has a characteristic notch in its motion immediately after the E point of the mitral valve in diastole. The distance between the septum and the anterior mitral leaflet at its point of closure is used to obtain an index of the size of the left ventricular outflow tract. Anterior to the septum is the echo-free chamber of the right ventricle.

The posterior mitral leaflet exhibits an opposing motion to the anterior mitral leaflet, making them appear as mirror images. Depending upon transducer angulation, the posterior wall of either the left ventricle or the left atrium will be seen posterior to the mitral leaflets. A helpful means of differentiating between these structures is observation of wall motion in relation to electrocardiographic timing. Near the mitral annulus, the left atrial posterior wall moves posteriorly during ventricular systole, just after the QRS complex. Conversely, the posterior wall of the left ventricle moves anteriorly in ventricular systole (Fig. 4–4).

As an aid in the identification and description of the various phases of mitral motion, early investigators assigned a letter to certain points of this motion, designated A, B, C, D, E, and F. The A wave occurs just after the P wave of the electrocardiogram (atrial systole) and occurs during atrial contraction. The A point generally is lower in amplitude than the E point and signifies the beginning of total mitral valve closure. Point B occurs at the beginning of ventricular contraction. This is followed by a rapid posterior movement that terminates at point C, the time of mitral closure and ordinarily the most posterior position of the mitral leaflets. This point occurs just after the QRS complex of the electrocardiogram. The left ventricle moves anteriorly with systole as a unit, and thus the echoes from the closed mitral leaflets move anteriorly from the C point to the D point at the end of systole. The line of normal mitral closure is frequently seen as multiple echoes instead of two clear, converging lines. These multiple echoes probably represent beam reflections from the chordae tendineae near their point of insertion as well as from the irregular surface of the leaflets. The same phenomenon can be seen in diastole for the same reason. True leaflet separation is observed just after the D point, when the two leaflets rapidly open to their maximal separation, the E point.[2-4] The E point is the most anterior position recorded during the cardiac cycle. There is then another period of posterior movement to point F, where both leaflets basically remain until late diastole (Fig. 4–5).

One of the most useful measurements of mitral valve motion is the diastolic descent rate (E-F slope). The E-F slope is a hemodynamic function of the duration of a positive gradient across the mitral valve and represents the rate of left atrial emptying and left ventricular filling during diastole.[5] It continues to be an important indicator of

mitral valve disease.[6-9] The most common use of this measurement is in the evaluation of adult patients with mitral stenosis who demonstrate a decreased slope. The E-F slope is also reduced when the compliance of the left ventricle is reduced, such as in idiopathic hypertrophic subaortic stenosis, hypertension, and aortic stenosis. It may be abnormally high in mitral insufficiency or in other conditions causing increased flow across the mitral valve. The E-F velocity is computed as a distance-time relationship, as shown in Figure 4–6.

The amplitude of excursion of the anterior mitral leaflet from point D to point E is a qualitative parameter of the flow across the valve, as well as of valve mobility. For example, the amplitude of movement is reduced in patients with thickening of the leaflets and shortening of the chordae tendineae.[10] The amplitude is measured from the D point to the level of the E point in a perpendicular line (Fig. 4–6).

RECORDING TECHNIQUE

Most of the major components of the heart can be recorded in the majority of patients. However, the mitral valve especially lends itself to this diagnostic modality for two reasons: first, its anatomical location makes it accessible to the ultrasound beam in over 90 per cent of adult patients; and second, the opening and closing motion of the mitral leaflets is directly parallel to the ultrasound beam. Consequently, the mitral valve is the most extensively studied of the cardiac valves, and many abnormalities of this valve are relatively easy to diagnose.

In the majority of cases, the fourth intercostal space, near the left sternal border, serves as the best position for transducer placement for detection of the mitral valve. The anatomical continuity of the posterior aortic root with the anterior mitral leaflet makes the aortic root an excellent choice as an echocardiographic landmark in the identification and recording of the mitral valve. Furthermore, the A-mode appearance of the parallel-moving double echoes of the aortic root is among the most characteristic of all patterns seen on the echocardiogram.

Following recognition of the aortic root on the A-mode display, slight angulation of the transducer inferiorly and laterally will reveal a change in the subtle motion of the

Text continued on page 48

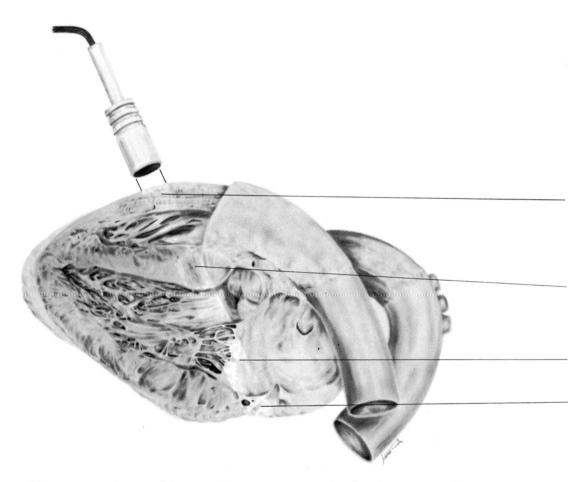

Figure 4–4. Ultrasound beam through the heart, viewed from the left lateral projection. Key: AWRV = anterior wall of the right ventricle; IVS = interventricular septum; MV = mitral valve; AML = anterior leaflet of the mitral valve; PML = posterior leaflet of the mitral valve; PW = posterior wall.

Illustration continued on opposite page

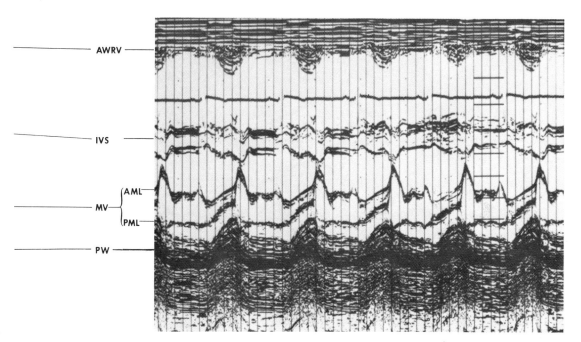

Figure 4-4   Continued.

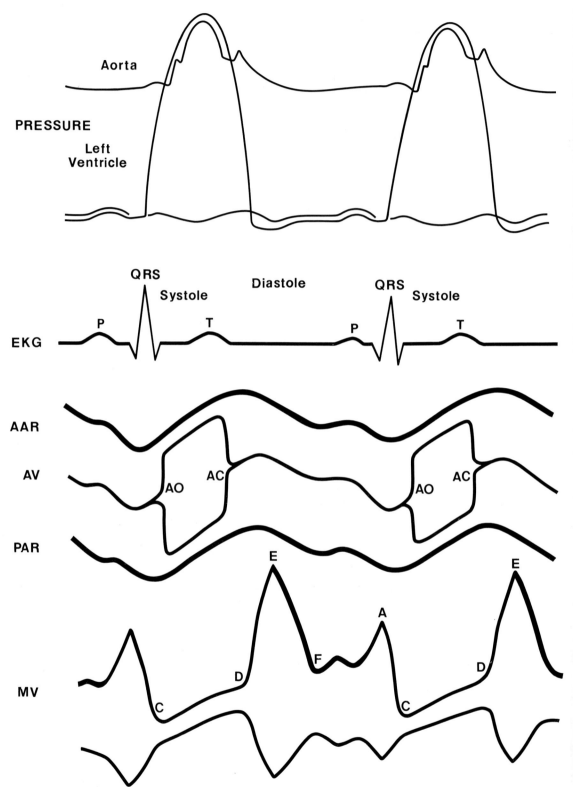

Figure 4–5. The phases of mitral motion are depicted relative to the pressure changes within the left atrium (LA) and left ventricle (LV). During systole, the mitral valve (MV) is closed, and the aortic valve (AV) opens (AO). At the end of systole, the aortic valve closes (AC), after which the mitral valve leaflets rapidly open to their maximum separation, the E point in early diastole (AAR = anterior aortic root; PAR = posterior aortic root).

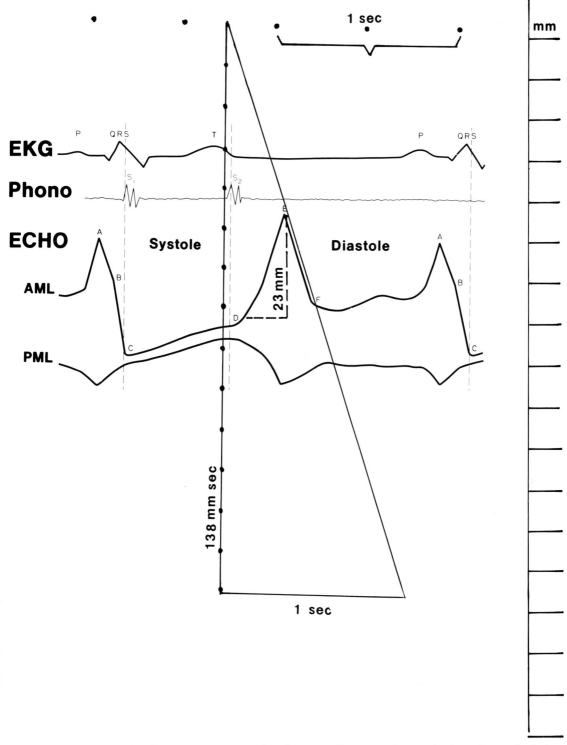

Figure 4-6. Mitral valve measurement. This diagram illustrates the method used in calculating the diastolic closing slope (E-F) and the maximal amplitude of the mitral leaflet. The diastolic descent rate of the mitral leaflet (E-F) is measured by extending its slope and determining the distance that it would descend in one second. The measurement of the amplitude of movement is the vertical distance from its closed position (D point) to its fully opened position (E point). In this normal valve, the diastolic descent rate is approximately 138 mm/sec, and the maximal amplitude is 23 mm (AML = anterior mitral leaflet; PML = posterior mitral leaflet).

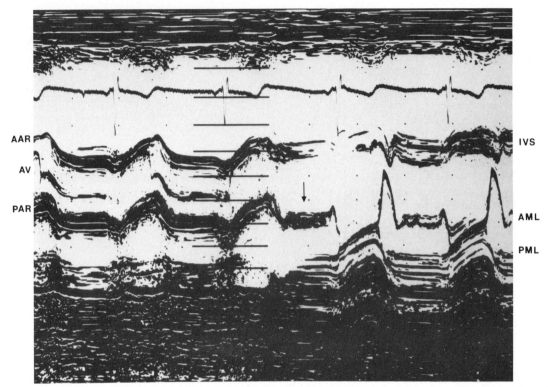

AAR
AV
PAR
IVS
AML
PML

Figure 4–7. Scan from the aortic root to the mitral valve. As the transducer is angled inferiorly and laterally from the aortic root, the anterior wall of the aortic root (AAR) is continuous with the septum (IVS), and the posterior wall of the aortic root (PAR) is continuous with the anterior mitral leaflet (AML) (arrow) (AV = aortic valve; PML = posterior mitral leaflet).

posterior aortic root to a "whip-like" motion representative of the anterior mitral valve leaflet. Simultaneously, the anterior wall of the aortic root will merge with the interventricular septum (Fig. 4–7). Angulation adjustment should continue until the echo representative of the anterior mitral leaflet is seen moving rapidly back and forth over a range of approximately 2 cm. When viewed on the A-mode, this dynamic range of motion often facilitates selection of the best transducer position. In front of, or anterior to, the anterior leaflet, there should be a relatively stationary group of echoes originating from the interventricular septum. At this time, the depth compensation (TGC) ramp should be adjusted to rest against the leading edge of the anterior septal wall. The near gain is then adjusted so that an echo-free space (the right ventricle) appears between the septal echo and the anterior chest wall echoes (see Figure 4–3).

While maintaining clear visualization of the anterior mitral leaflet, slight angulation of the transducer more inferiorly and later-ally should allow for visualization of the posterior leaflet. It will move in a similar but opposite pattern to the anterior leaflet. Precise transducer angulation becomes more critical as the ultrasound beam approaches this area, mainly because the posterior mitral leaflet provides a smaller target for the echo beam, and its motion is much less extensive when compared to that of the anterior leaflet (see Figure 4–4). It should be emphasized that most measurements and descriptions of mitral motion are best made when the valve is recorded at the point of its maximum excursion, when both leaflets are visualized. Directing the transducer too inferiorly or superiorly will result in factitious reduction of mitral motion (Figs. 4–8 and 4–9).

With respect to the M-mode presentation, it is usually necessary to make additional fine control adjustments, such as gain or reject, prior to actual recording. To accurately assess leaflet thickness, some of the low-gain echoes must be removed. In the event of suspected leaflet calcification, the inten-

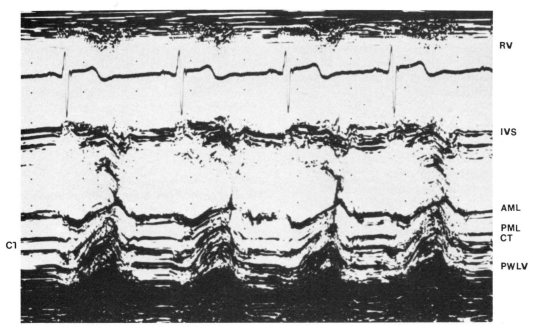

Figure 4-8. Directing the transducer too inferiorly produces reduced mitral motion. In this view, the ultrasound beam is being directed more toward the posterior mitral leaflet (PML). The anterior mitral leaflet (AML) has a "smudged" appearance. The chordae tendineae (CT) and the mitral leaflets appear as multi-layered lines. Note the poor definition of septal (IVS) motion (RV = right ventricle; PWLV = posterior wall of the left ventricle).

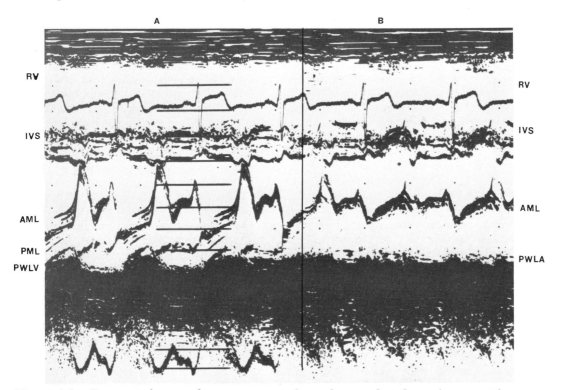

Figure 4-9. Directing the transducer too superiorly produces reduced mitral motion. The section designated A demonstrates maximal mitral motion with good visualization of the posterior mitral leaflet (PML). The section designated B demonstrates a marked reduction of the anterior mitral leaflet (AML), and the posterior mitral leaflet is not seen. This is due to the ultrasound beam striking a position near the aorta. Note the contraction of the posterior wall of the left ventricle (PWLV) in section A versus that of the posterior wall of the left atrium (PWLA) in section B (RV = right ventricle; IVS = interventricular septum).

sity of the echoes can be compared with that of a neighboring structure such as the interventricular septum or the posterior wall of the left ventricle.

VARIATIONS AND DISEASES OF THE MITRAL VALVE

There are many conditions that produce a variation in the appearance of the mitral valve. These are divided into two main classifications: (1) abnormalities involving other structures within the heart that secondarily affect the function and appearance of the normal mitral valve and (2) disease of the valve apparatus or the leaflets themselves.

Cardiac Arrhythmias

Alterations of cardiac rhythm can have profound effects on the appearance of the normal mitral valve.[11, 12] This is discussed in depth in Chapter 3 ("The Electrocardiogram and the Echocardiogram").

Edler, in his classic echocardiographic studies of the mitral valve,[11] showed that a distinct A wave is not present in atrial fibrillation, presumably because synchronous atrial contraction does not occur. On these recordings, the mitral valve leaflets usually exhibit small-amplitude opening and closing movements for the duration of diastole. Occasionally, single high-amplitude openings resembling the normal A wave are seen late in diastole (Figs. 4–10 and 4–11). The mitral valve in atrial flutter may be observed to have regular, low-amplitude diastolic excursions that coincide with the flutter waves on the electrocardiogram. The diastolic oscillations of the mitral valve seen in patients with atrial fibrillation and atrial flutter are more pronounced and are of a lower frequency than the fine diastolic oscillations seen in patients with aortic regurgitation.

In sinus tachycardia, the "M" configuration of the anterior mitral leaflet is lost, as diastole shortens and the E and A waves merge, causing the valve to have a single opening (Figs. 4–12 to 4–14).[13]

Conditions that prolong the P-R interval of the electrocardiogram, such as extreme first degree heart block, will also produce a single opening of the valve (Fig. 4–15).[2]

Variations in normal mitral valve motion also occur as a result of premature contractions. For example, in the presence of premature atrial contractions, the E-A mitral interval shortens during the diastolic period following the premature beat. During the longer diastolic period after the premature beat, the E-A interval is correspondingly longer. In subjects with premature ventricular beats, closure of the mitral valve occurs early, usually without a preceding A wave. With marked prematurity of ventricular contraction, the mitral valve may be prevented from opening at all (Fig. 4–16).[2]

In view of the many variations of mitral valve motion that occur as a result of cardiac arrhythmias, every echocardiogram should include a simultaneous electrocardiogram. The QRS complex of the electrocardiogram also serves as a fixed reference point within each cardiac cycle from which the individual cardiac structures can be timed.

Ventricular Compliance

The left ventricle is by far the dominant of the two left heart chambers in terms of the internal pressures generated. Thus, the motion of a normal mitral valve may be assumed to be primarily a manifestation of left ventricular pressure and volume. For example, when the end-systolic pressure within the left ventricle is markedly increased, the mitral valve may open only in late diastole following atrial contraction, giving it the appearance of a single opening valve (Fig. 4–17).[14]

The normal diastolic descent (E-F) slope of the anterior mitral valve leaflet can appear markedly decreased in the presence of slow left ventricular filling. As the left ventricular compliance decreases, as occurs in the myocardial infiltrative diseases,[15] left ventricular hypertrophy, and coronary disease,[16] the flow rate across the mitral valve decreases. Hemodynamically, the rate of diastolic closure of the anterior mitral leaflet is dependent on two factors: (1) the duration of a positive gradient across the valve and (2) the rate of left ventricular filling during diastole.[3] Consequently, with decreased ventricular compliance, the mitral valve maintains a longer period of opening during diastole to accommodate the slower flow rate into the "stiff" ventricle. In these diseased states, reduced left ventricular

Text continued on page 57

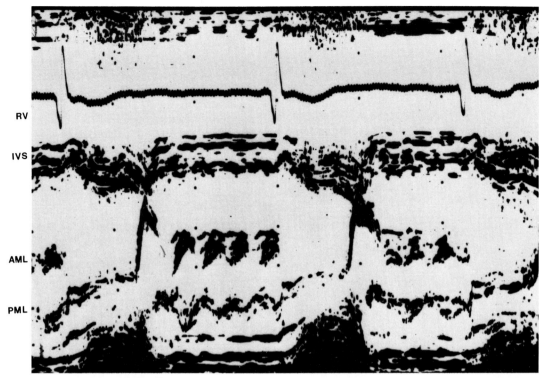

Figure 4–10. Atrial fibrillation and mitral motion. Pronounced undulations are seen during the diastolic opening of the mitral valve. It is of interest to note that these diastolic undulations are reflected in both the anterior mitral leaflet (AML) and the posterior mitral leaflet (PML) (RV = right ventricle; IVS = interventricular septum).

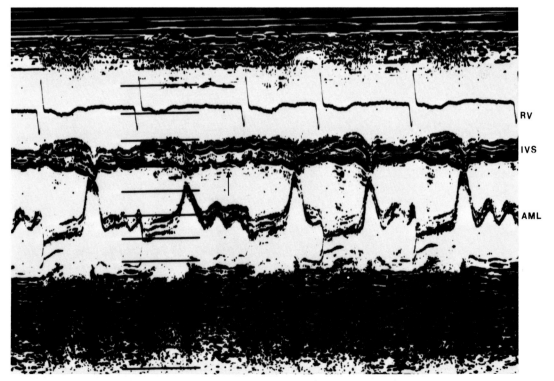

Figure 4–11. Atrial fibrillation. During diastole, both the anterior mitral leaflet (AML) and the interventricular septum (IVS) exhibit an undulating motion (arrow) (RV = right ventricle).

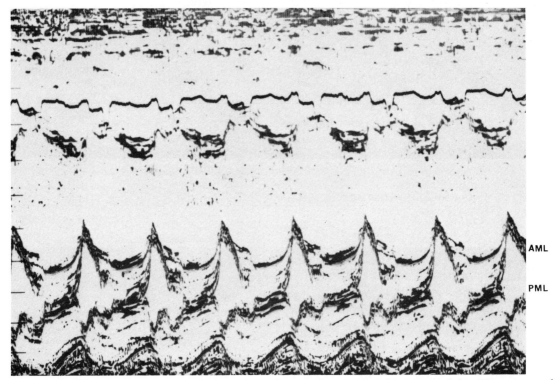

Figure 4–12.   Mitral motion in sinus tachycardia. The normal configuration of the anterior mitral leaflet (AML) is lost as diastole is shortened, causing the anterior leaflet to have only one opening with only a brief A wave. The posterior mitral leaflet (PML) shows a normal motion. The overall "shaggy" appearance of this valve is due to mitral leaflet vegetation from infective endocarditis.

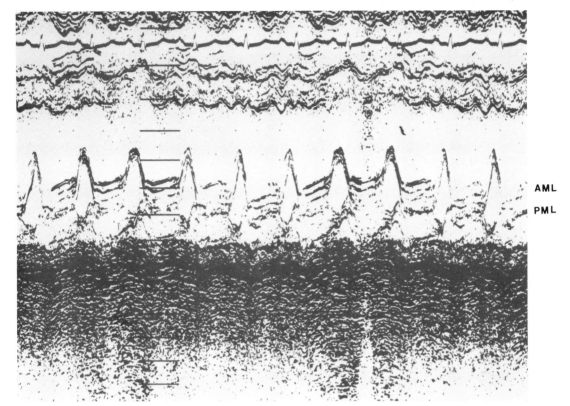

Figure 4–13. The single opening valve in supraventricular tachycardia. As a result of the rapid heart rate, the E and A waves of the anterior mitral leaflet (AML) have merged. Upon close observation it is of interest to note that the posterior mitral leaflet (PML) exhibits a normal double opening.

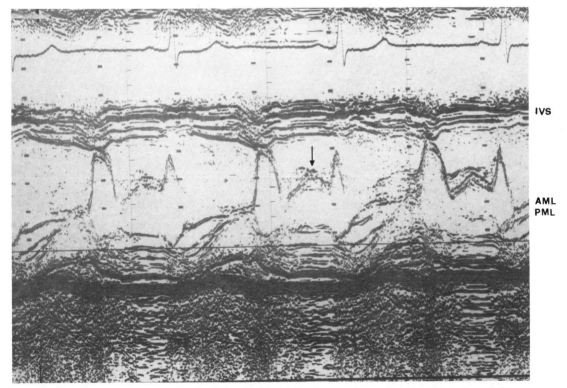

Figure 4–14. Mitral motion in sinus bradycardia. In the presence of a slow heart rate (45 beats per minute), it is not an abnormal finding to visualize a pronounced hump in the mid-diastolic phase of normal mitral motion (arrow). The mitral valve may also open wider during the interval between the two anterior deflections (AML = anterior mitral leaflet; PML = posterior mitral leaflet; IVS = interventricular septum).

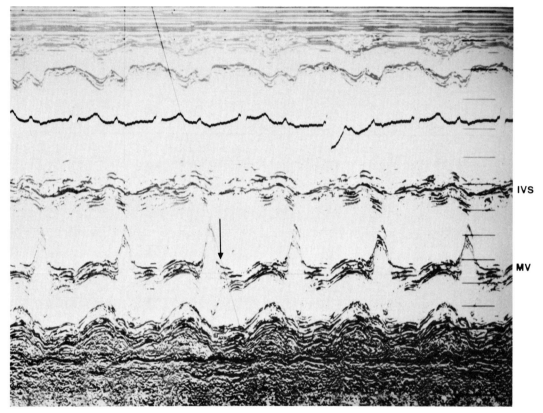

IVS

MV

Figure 4–15.   The single-opening mitral valve in first-degree heart block. Echocardiographically, the mitral valve (MV) in first-degree heart block is characterized by the absence of the A wave (arrow). As a result of atrial contraction occurring early, the A wave is fused with the E wave, and mitral closure is premature (arrow) (IVS = interventricular septum).

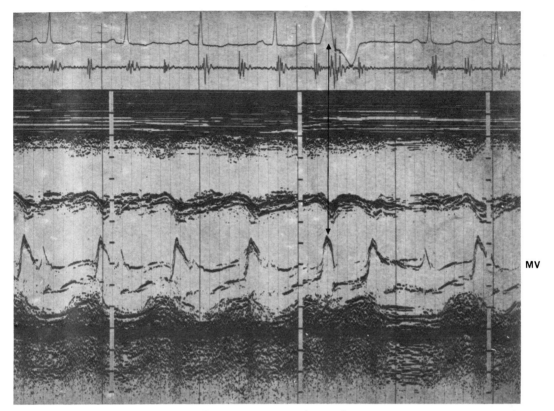

Figure 4–16. Premature ventricular contraction and mitral motion. A premature ventricular contraction (arrow) causes early closure of the mitral valve (MV).

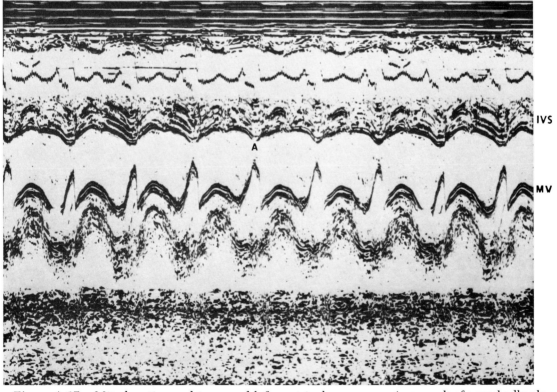

Figure 4–17. Mitral motion and increased left ventricular pressure. As a result of a markedly elevated left ventricular end-systolic pressure, the mitral E point, representing mitral opening in early diastole, is absent. Following atrial contraction, the mitral valve (MV) exhibits a single opening (A wave) (IVS = interventricular septum).

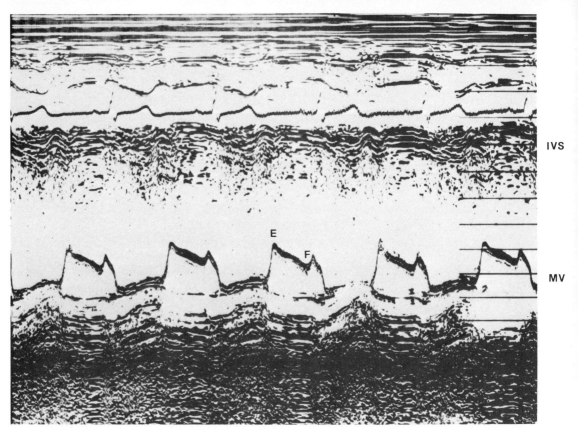

IVS

MV

E

F

Figure 4–18. Mitral motion and reduced left ventricular compliance. The mitral diastolic descent rate (E-F) is diminished to approximately 20 mm/sec as a result of the decreased flow to the left ventricle (IVS = interventricular septum).

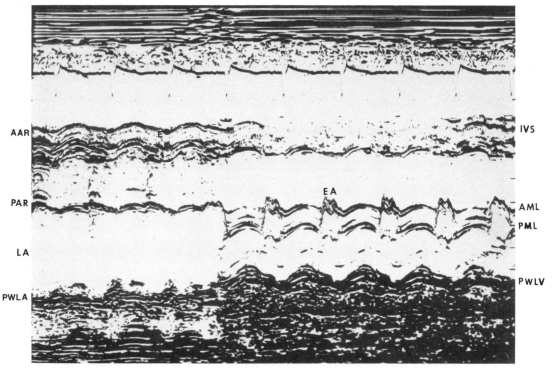

AAR

PAR

LA

PWLA

IVS

AML

PML

PWLV

E

EA

Figure 4–19. The mitral valve in left ventricular failure. In this scan from the aorta to the mitral valve, the opening amplitude (D-E) is markedly reduced. The E and A waves are equally reduced in amplitude. The entire mitral apparatus is displaced from the posterior wall of the left ventricle (PWLV) (AML = anterior mitral leaflet; PML = posterior mitral leaflet; IVS = interventricular septum; AAR = anterior aortic root; PAR = posterior aortic root; LA = left atrium; PWLA = posterior wall of the left atrium).

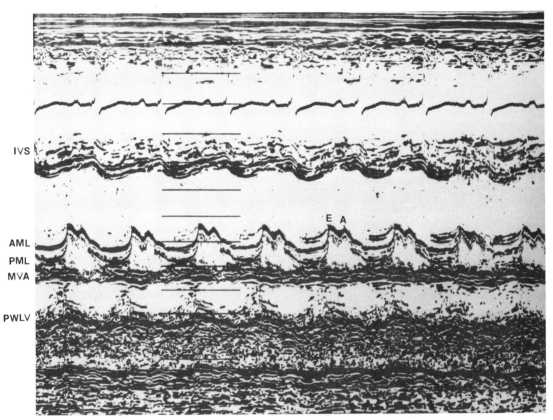

IVS

AML
PML
MVA

PWLV

E A

Figure 4–20.   Restricted mitral motion in left ventricular failure. As the flow into the left ventricle is restricted, the amplitude of the mitral leaflet is markedly reduced. Although the anterior mitral leaflet (AML) exhibits diminished motion, the posterior mitral leaflet (PML) is partially masked by the thickened mitral valve annulus (MVA). The E and A waves are nearly identical in amplitude (IVS = interventricular septum; PWLV = posterior wall of the left ventricle).

compliance may therefore be manifested on the echocardiogram as a diminished E-F slope.

In some instances, the E-F slope can be so slow as to simulate the condition of mitral stenosis (Figs. 4–18 to 4–20).

Left Atrial Tumors

In the presence of a left atrial myxoma, the mitral valve assumes the following characteristics:[17-21]

1. Blunted E point.
2. Reduced E-F slope.
3. The recording of the valve tissue itself may be poorly separated from the heavy band of echoes from the tumor immediately adjacent.
4. There is usually a slight delay from the time of valve opening until the tumor echoes appear (Fig. 4–21).

The echocardiographic detection of a left atrial myxoma is principally contingent upon the tumor's extending through the mitral orifice during mitral valve opening.[22, 23] Such protrusion probably occurs in the majority of cases. The technologist who is not informed of the possibility of a myxoma or who is unfamiliar with its echocardiographic appearance may make an effort to "clean up" these echoes by reducing the echo intensity to the point at which the tumor echoes are poorly recorded. Conversely, in the presence of severe mitral valve calcification, it is possible to produce false positives by adjusting the gain to such an extent that the echoes are dramatically magnified (Fig. 4–22). The diagnosis will also be missed if the tumor is not traversing the mitral orifice at the time of the examination, although sometimes the tumor can be seen within the left atrium. When the diagnosis of a myxoma is suspected, long, uninterrupted recordings of the mitral valve with the patient in various positions may be

AML

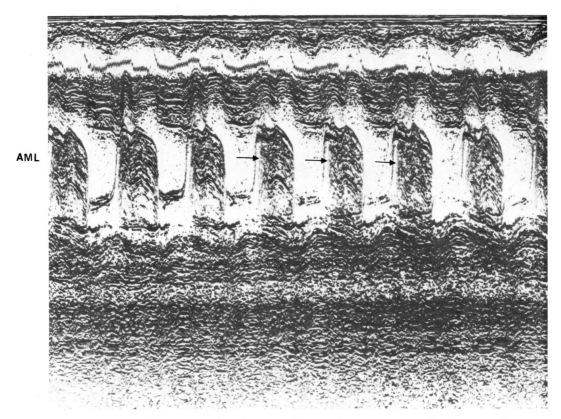

Figure 4–21.   Left atrial myxoma. The cluster of dense echoes seen immediately behind the ante-rior mitral leaflet (AML) originate from the tumor as it protrudes through the mitral orifice during opening (diastole). Note the slight delay from the time of valve opening until the tumor echoes appear (arrows).

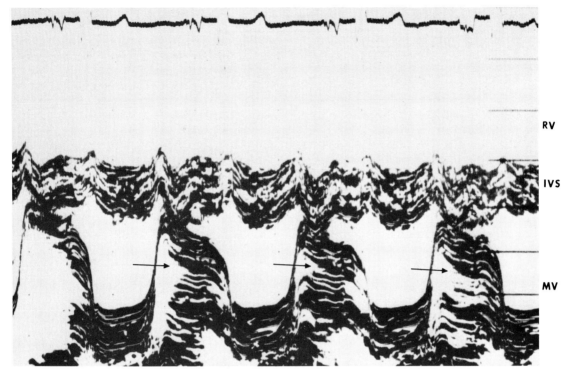

Figure 4–22. The presence of marked calcification of the mitral leaflets bears a resemblance to a protruding left atrial tumor (arrows) (RV = right ventricle; IVS = interventricular septum; MV = mitral valve).

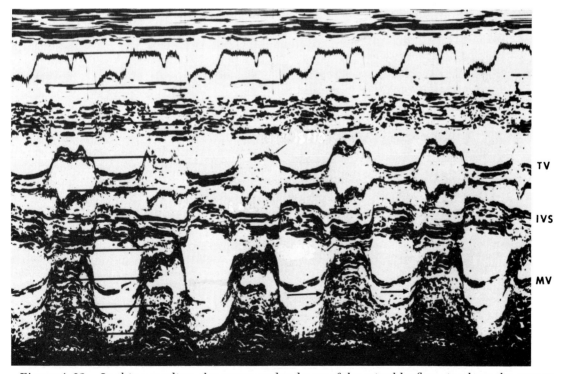

Figure 4–23. In this recording, the severe redundancy of the mitral leaflets simulates the appearance of a mass (arrows). The tricuspid valve (TV) is clearly seen as a result of pulmonary hypertension (IVS = interventricular septum; MV = mitral valve).

necessary to confirm or deny the presence of a tumor. When the index of suspicion is high and echocardiographic results are negative, repeat examinations may be warranted (Fig. 4–23).

Idiopathic Hypertrophic Subaortic Stenosis (IHSS)

In IHSS, the mitral valve is often abnormal, and several echocardiographic anomalies are now well recognized (Fig. 4–24).[24-29] This condition is characterized by asymmetric hypertrophy of the interventricular septum and consequent narrowing of the left ventricular outflow tract. Obstruction of the left ventricular outflow tract is produced during mid-systole by the anterior mitral leaflet as it moves toward the interventricular septum. Simultaneously with the outflow obstruction, there is sometimes mitral regurgitation, which is also produced by the abnormal anterior motion of the anterior leaflet. There is also reduction of inflow due to the noncompliant left ventricle. The echocardiographic features of the mitral valve are as follows:

1. Reduced E-F slope secondary to reduced left ventricular compliance.

2. Narrowing of the outflow tract. The mitral valve may strike the septum in diastole.

3. Mid-systolic excursion of the anterior leaflet of the mitral valve toward the septum with return before diastole.

In severe IHSS, the aortic valve may open rapidly several times during one cardiac cycle as the anterior motion (SAM) obstructs flow. The obstruction produces a variation of flow through the valve, causing it to open and close, open and close (Fig. 4–25).

In many cases of IHSS, the mitral valve is surprisingly difficult to record. This is probably because of its restricted amplitude of motion and the fact that it appears to be

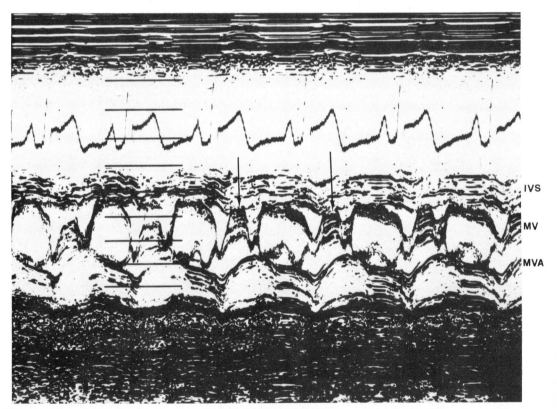

Figure 4–24. The mitral valve in idiopathic hypertrophic subaortic stenosis. The abnormal anterior motion of the anterior mitral leaflet during systole is probably the most characteristic echocardiographic finding in this pathology (arrows). Note that both the abrupt anterior systolic motion and the anterior mitral leaflet strike the septum (IVS) (MV = mitral valve; MVA = mitral valve annulus).

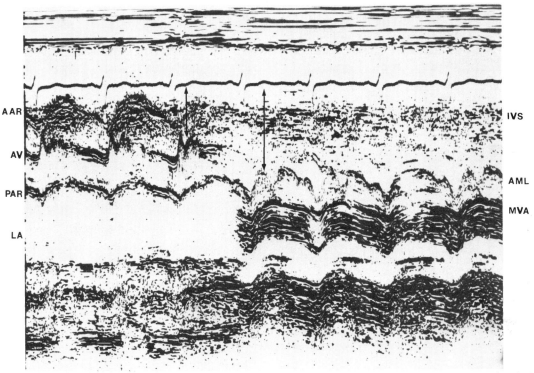

Figure 4–25. The aortic valve in idiopathic hypertrophic subaortic stenosis. The aortic valve (AV) exhibits a premature closure in mid-systole (arrow), reopens, and closes again in end-systole. The initial premature closure of the aortic valve occurs at the same time (mid-systole) as the anterior mitral leaflet (AML) exhibits its abrupt abnormal anterior motion (arrow) (AAR = anterior aortic root; PAR = posterior aortic root; LA = left atrium; IVS = interventricular septum). Note the abnormally thickened mitral valve annulus (MVA).

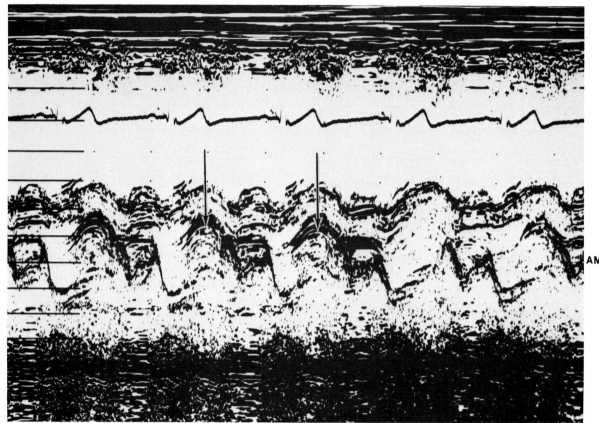

AML

Figure 4–26. Incorrect transducer angulation simulating idiopathic hypertrophic subaortic stenosis. A "pseudo" anterior motion of the anterior mitral leaflet (AML) during systole is produced by the superimposition of a portion of the posterior wall of the aortic root (arrows).

squeezed between the thickened interventricular septum and the posterior left ventricular wall.

Transducer angulation is critical and should be executed in such a manner that the ultrasound beam strikes a position nearer to the tip of the leaflet. It is here that the largest systolic anterior movement can be observed. In the event that the transducer is tilted too posteriorly toward the proximal portions of the valve, the systolic movement of the valve will be retarded. In addition, when aiming the transducer more toward the base of the valve, the leaflet may possibly exhibit no systolic abnormality. Scanning slowly from the aortic root to the mitral valve is an excellent means of observing any abnormal systolic motion, mainly because the ultrasound beam will first strike a position nearer to the tip of the leaflet. At the same time, caution must be exercised in the event that a "pseudo IHSS" pattern be created by the superimposition of the posterior aortic root echo on that of the mitral

valve leaflet (Fig. 4–26). Minute angulations of the transducer should be a continuous process until the valve and its anatomical relationships are clearly delineated. It must also be emphasized that too little gain or too much attenuation can fail to demonstrate any abnormal systolic movement and, just as importantly, give an incorrect recording as to the true thickness of the interventricular septum and left ventricular wall.

Occasionally, although IHSS is suspected, the abnormal systolic motion may be latent. In this event, administration of amyl nitrite by the physician can produce the recognizable abnormality and permit the echocardiographic visualization of the otherwise latent or intermittent condition.[30]

Papillary Muscle Dysfunction

Under normal circumstances, papillary muscle contraction occurring simultaneously with left ventricular contraction is thought to tense the chordae tendineae, thereby preventing prolapse of the leaflets into the left atrium. Normal chordal tension may not be maintained during ventricular systole by an intact papillary muscle under the following conditions: (1) abnormal papillary muscle contraction, a common occurrence in coronary artery disease; (2) adjacent myocardial wall dysfunction, i.e., infarction or fibrosis; (3) left ventricular dilatation; and (4) ruptured chordae tendineae.

While coronary disease is probably the most common cause of papillary muscle dysfunction, other conditions such as cardiomyopathy and myocardial infiltrative diseases may cause this syndrome both by direct papillary muscle involvement and by disease of the adjacent left ventricular wall.[2]

Severe left ventricular dilatation causes a displacement of the papillary muscle to a more distant position from the mitral leaflets. This may prohibit normal conformity of the mitral leaflets during ventricular systole.[2, 31-33]

The dominant echocardiographic features of papillary muscle dysfunction include: (1) a blunted mitral valve E point, probably due to reduced left ventricular compliance and (2) slight fluttering of the anterior leaflet of the mitral valve during diastole, caused by failure of the chordae to maintain tension when the leaflets are in their open position. When the left ventricle is large, similar fluttering is seen, and in the case of left ventricular failure, the typical low-flow diamond-shaped appearance is seen (Figs. 4–27 and 4–28). (See also Figure 4–20). Differentiation of the leaflet fluttering due to papillary muscle dysfunction from aortic regurgitation is difficult to diagnose solely from the echocardiographic recording, necessitating other clinical information in most cases.

Mitral Valve Prolapse

Normally, both the anterior and posterior leaflets of the mitral valve come together in early systole and stay together throughout systole, during which time there is a gradual anterior motion of both leaflets. The motion

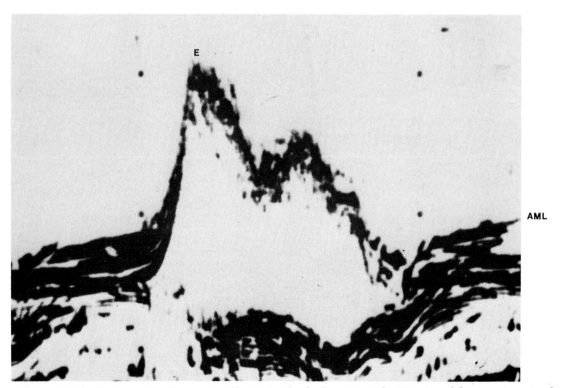

Figure 4–27.   The mitral valve in papillary muscle dysfunction. The E point of the anterior mitral leaflet (AML) is blunted, and there is gross fluttering of the leaflet throughout the cardiac cycle.

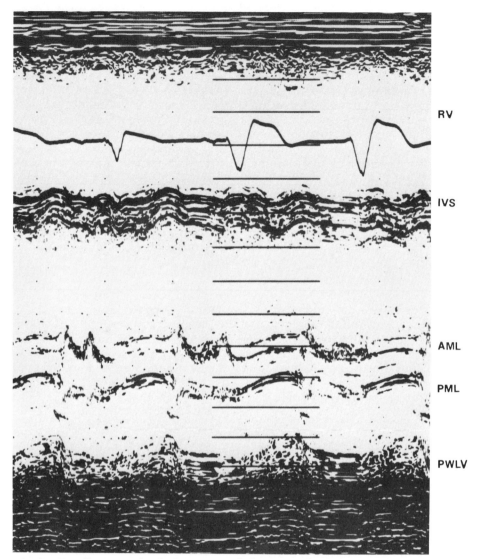

Figure 4–28. Papillary muscle dysfunction in left ventricular failure. There is gross fluttering of both the anterior mitral leaflet (AML) and the posterior mitral leaflet (PML). The entire mitral apparatus is displaced from the posterior wall of the left ventricle (PWLV) (RV = right ventricle; IVS = interventricular septum).

of the normal mitral leaflets and that during mitral leaflet prolapse are similar during diastole. The diastolic motion of leaflets that prolapse is normal. However, during ventricular systole one or both leaflets exhibit an abnormal posterior protrusion into the left atrium.

Mitral prolapse has been described under various names, including "Barlow's syndrome,"[34] "floppy valve syndrome," "systolic click–late systolic murmur syndrome," and "billowed[35] or ballooned mitral valve."[36]

In most cases of mitral valve prolapse, the condition does not progress to significant clinical deterioration, although several complications have been described, including: (1) mitral regurgitation;[37, 38] (2) bacterial endocarditis;[37] (3) serious arrhythmias;[39 40] (4) chordal rupture;[37, 41] and (5) sudden death.[42, 43]

When either or both of the mitral leaflets appear to move posteriorly at any point after the C point of the mitral valve, prolapse into the atrium must be suspected. It should be emphasized that it is sometimes not clear

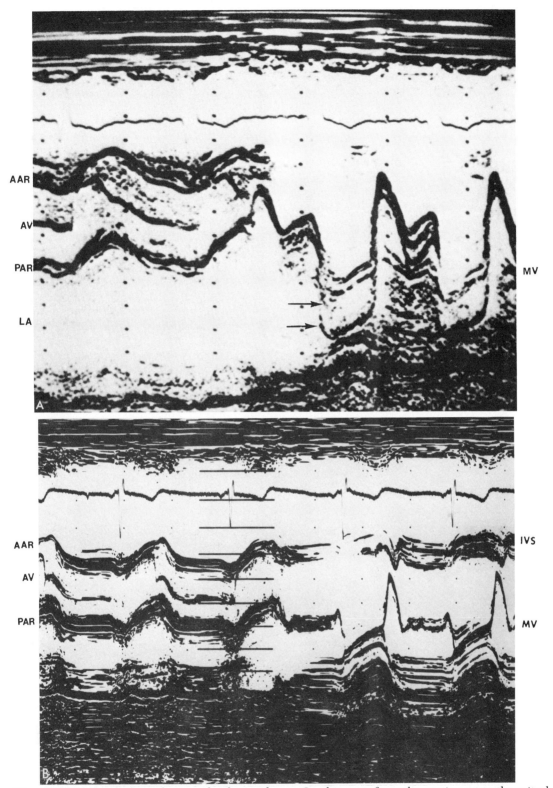

Figure 4-29. (A) Pansystolic mitral valve prolapse. On this scan from the aortic root to the mitral valve (MV), the mitral leaflet echoes are markedly displaced toward the area of the left atrium (LA) during ventricular systole (arrows). The left atrium (LA) is dilated as a result of associated mitral regurgitation (AAR = anterior aortic root; AV = aortic valve; PAR = posterior aortic root). (B) Normal mitral leaflet placement on this scan from the aortic root to the mitral valve (AAR = anterior aortic root; AV = aortic valve; PAR = posterior aortic root; IVS = interventricular septum; MV = mitral valve).

from the echocardiogram which of the two leaflets is prolapsing. Prolapse of the anterior leaflet, however, is usually easier to identify than prolapse of the posterior leaflet, mainly because it is the easiest leaflet to record.

Mitral prolapse can be especially appreciated when scanning from the aortic root to the mitral valve (Fig. 4–29). Normally, the anterior mitral leaflet moves no more than a few millimeters beyond the most posterior excursion of the aortic posterior wall. When the anterior leaflet appears to move as far posteriorly as the left atrial wall during systole, this may be regarded as strong evidence for prolapse. Scanning *slowly* back and forth from the aortic root to the mitral valve is particularly important, because it is possible to create a false positive mitral valve prolapse by abrupt transducer change from aortic root to mitral valve. A continuous sweep from the left ventricle to the mitral valve and aortic root frequently facilitates recognition of true prolapse, probably because this technique requires the operator to make very gradual transducer changes

(Fig. 4–30). False positives can also be obtained by placing the transducer too high on the chest and directing it too inferiorly (Fig. 4–31).[44] Early systolic plunges of the mitral leaflets, with rapid recovery or flattening of the leaflets in systole, can be technically produced and should not be considered reliable indicators of prolapse. Furthermore, simple failure of the two leaflets to appear to come together during systole ordinarily cannot be considered representative of true leaflet separation.

In cases where the valve leaflets appear as multiple parallel lines during systole, it is often difficult to identify which is anterior and which is posterior, because of the redundancy of the leaflets. Quite often in these instances, the mitral-aortic sweep will be helpful in determining which leaflet is anterior and which is posterior. It should be mentioned that while clinical diagnosis of mitral valve prolapse has emphasized the posterior leaflet, echocardiographic studies have demonstrated that both leaflets are usually involved.

Prolapse of the mitral valve can be clas-

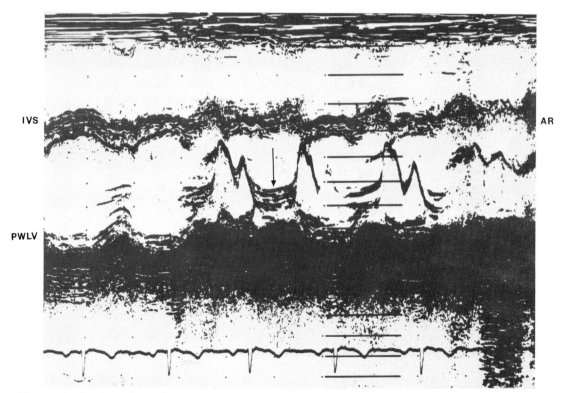

Figure 4–30.   Scan from the posterior wall of the left ventricle (PWLV) to the aortic root. As the transducer is slightly angled superiorly and medially from the left ventricle, the mitral valve leaflets exhibit a marked posterior displacement during ventricular systole, indicative of a pansystolic prolapse (arrow) (IVS = interventricular septum; AR = aortic root).

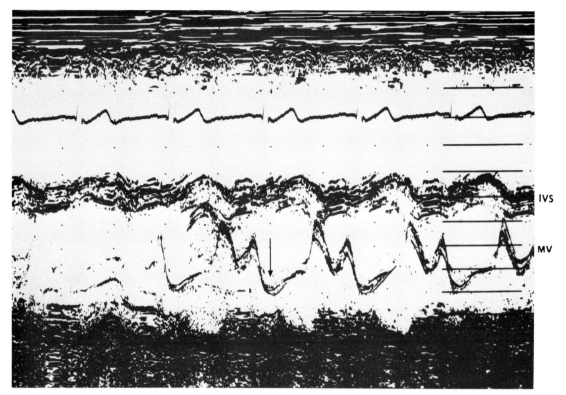

IVS

MV

Figure 4–31. Technical error simulating mitral prolapse. The "pseudo" posterior displacement of the valve leaflets in systole (arrow) is produced by placing the transducer too high on the chest and directing it too inferiorly. Note the overall unclarity of this recording and the exaggerated septal (IVS) motion, an important clue of incorrect transducer angulation (MV = mitral valve).

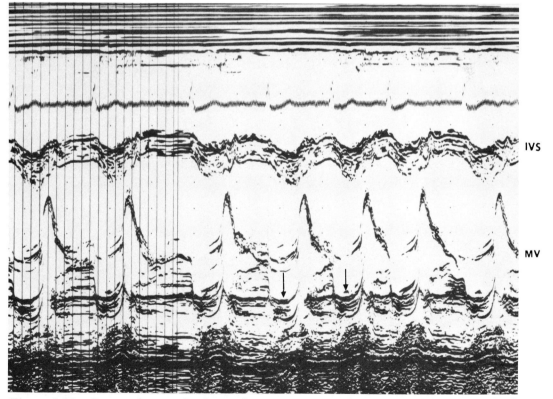

IVS

MV

Figure 4–32. Pansystolic mitral valve prolapse. During systole, portions of the anterior leaflet are buried within the posterior leaflet. Note the pronounced "hammock" effect of the leaflets throughout much of systole (arrows) (IVS = interventricular septum; MV = mitral valve).

sified into two distinct but often overlapping types, pansystolic and mid-systolic. A characteristic finding is a "hammock-like" or marked sagging motion of the leaflets posteriorly, with considerable leaflet separation during systole (Figs. 4–29A, 4–30, and 4–32).[45] DeMaria et al. found pansystolic prolapse to be the more common form.[46] There are cases in this type of prolapse when the leaflet echoes may actually become buried within the posterior wall echoes or will appear as multiple, parallel systolic echoes. This echo configuration probably results from the redundant layers of the abnormal leaflet structure, with each layer presenting a reflecting surface for the ultrasound beam (Fig. 4–32).[47]

The most obvious echocardiographic finding with mid-systolic prolapse is a step-like posterior motion of either one or both leaflets in systole replacing the normal gradual anterior systolic movement. The degree of posterior displacement depends in part upon the severity of the condition (Fig. 4–33). Occurring with the posterior displacement, a systolic click can usually be detected upon auscultation. This click is caused by either a sudden tensing of the prolapsed leaflet or abrupt tightening of the chordae tendineae.[2, 48]

In some patients, the findings of mitral valve prolapse may be intermittent (as the murmur may also be). Amyl nitrite inhalation[38, 49] may be useful in these cases. Inhalation of amyl nitrite causes an increase in venous pooling, and the end-diastolic volume of the left ventricle becomes diminished, conceivably leaving the leaflets nearer to a position of prolapse at end-diastole.[2] Fontana et al. have found that the upright posture decreases venous return and end-diastolic left ventricular volume.[50] Thus, it is useful to make echocardiographic recordings in both the upright and the reclining positions in patients in whom prolapse is suspected.

In some cases of severe prolapse, a mass of echoes resembling a protruding atrial tumor appears behind the mitral valve echo in diastole (Fig. 4–34). These echoes probably are reflected from layers of redundant valve tissue.

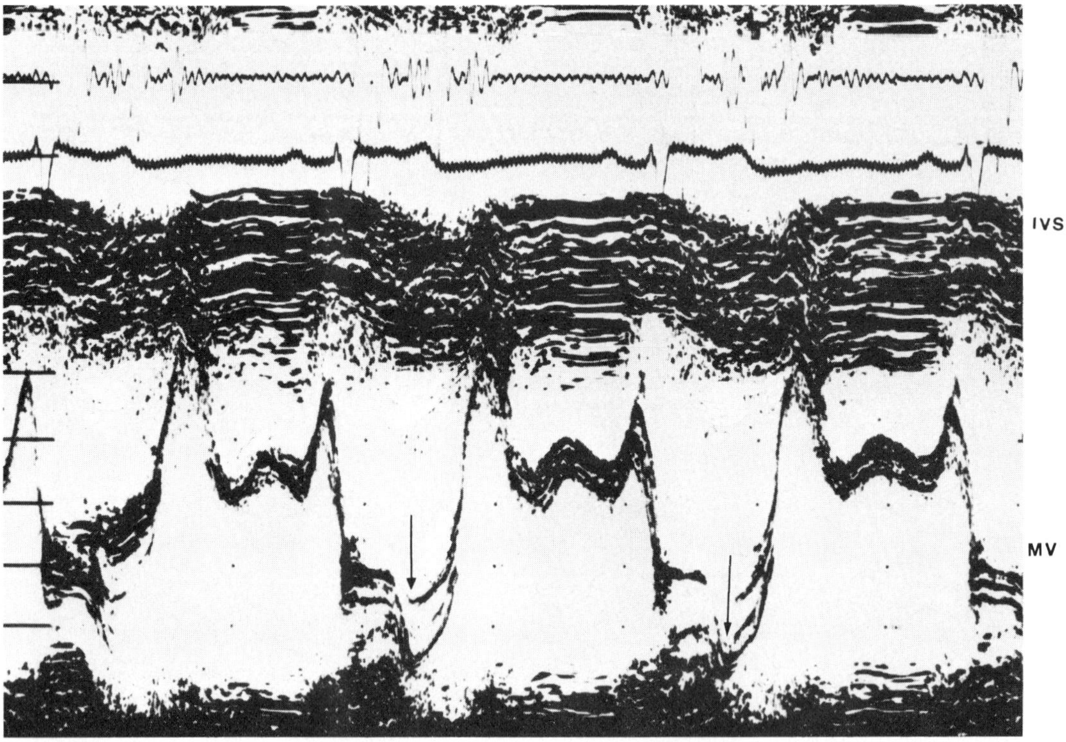

Figure 4–33. Mid-systolic mitral valve prolapse. Immediately after closure, the mitral leaflets begin their normal anterior excursion. In mid-systole, however, this motion is interrupted by a pronounced posterior displacement (arrows). Although both leaflets prolapse the posterior mitral leaflet is more severely displaced (arrow) (IVS = interventricular septum; MV = mitral valve).

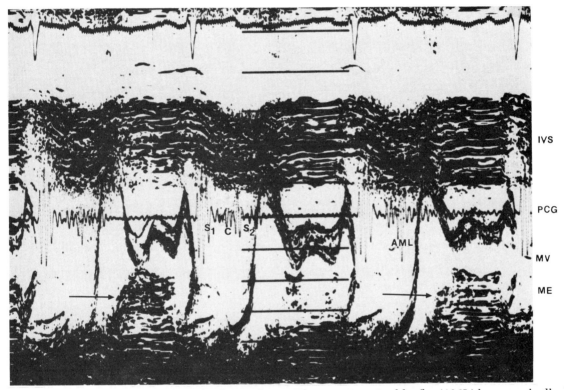

Figure 4–34.   Mid-systolic mitral valve prolapse. The anterior mitral leaflet (AML) has a markedly increased amplitude of excursion in excess of 40 mm. During valve opening (diastole), multiple echoes (ME) originating from the redundant valve tissue are seen (arrow). Recorded on the phonocardiogram (PCG), a click (C) is noted between the first heart sound (S_1) and the second heart sound (S_2) (IVS = interventricular septum; MV = mitral valve).

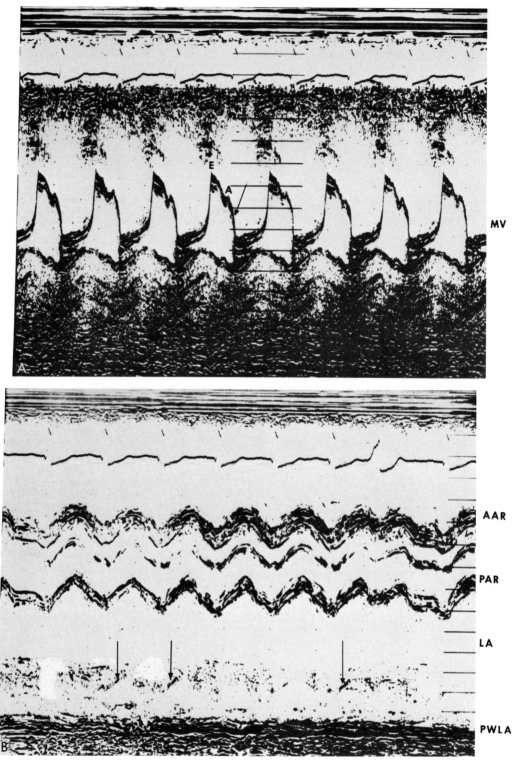

Figure 4-35. (A) Acute chordal rupture. The mitral valve (MV) exhibits an increased amplitude of excursion in excess of 30 mm, with coarse fluttering of the anterior leaflet (E point). Note the abrupt posterior plunge of the anterior leaflet following the A wave (arrow). (B) Recording of the same patient. In this view through the left atrium (LA), a portion of the posterior mitral leaflet appears during ventricular systole (arrows). On postmortem examination, the posterior mitral leaflet was totally flail and was lying in the left atrium. The left atrium is dilated (AAR = anterior aortic root; PAR = posterior aortic root; PWLA = posterior wall of the left atrium).

A simultaneous high-frequency apex phonocardiogram will usually help in the confirmation of a suspected echocardiographic appearance of prolapse (Fig. 4–34).

Ruptured Chordae Tendineae

Total severance of the chordae tendineae results in a marked alteration of mitral valve motion.[51, 52] It may occur either as an acute isolated event or as a result of multiple causes that are usually long-standing before the rupture occurs.[2, 53-55] Because chordal rupture is generally acute, the usual echocardiographic signs of mitral regurgitation, i.e., dilatation of the left atrium and left ventricle, are absent.[2]

Posterior leaflet chordal rupture has been recognized by a holosystolic posterior displacement (secondary prolapse) and by chaotic, anterior movements during diastole. In some cases, the leaflet of the corresponding ruptured chordae prolapses into the left atrium and appears as a fleeting echo within the left atrium during ventricular systole (Fig. 4–35).[56, 57]

Anterior leaflet involvement may appear as a coarse fluttering of the leaflet during systole. Because of the increased flow across the mitral valve, the anterior leaflet will show a greatly exaggerated opening excursion (Fig. 4–36).

Chronic Aortic Insufficiency

Aortic insufficiency can produce a variety of abnormal changes in the appearance of the normal mitral valve echo. The most obvious characteristic in chronic aortic insufficiency is the presence of a fine, rapid fluttering of the anterior mitral valve leaflet. This fluttering usually begins at the point of maximal opening (E point) and generally terminates with ventricular systole. This gives the anterior mitral leaflet a "sawtoothed" appearance as opposed to the smooth diastolic motion of the anterior leaflet when aortic insufficiency is not present. This fluttering is thought to originate from the regurgitant jet of the incompetent aortic valve.[58] The regurgitant jet may strike both mitral leaflets or the interventricular septum or all three.[59] This results in the phe-

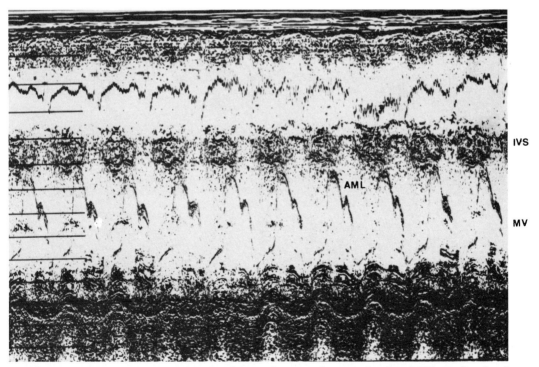

Figure 4–36. Acute rupture of the chordae tendineae. The mitral valve (MV) amplitude of excursion measures approximately 38 mm. Note the fine fluttering of the anterior mitral leaflet (AML) as it appears to be flung toward the septum (IVS).

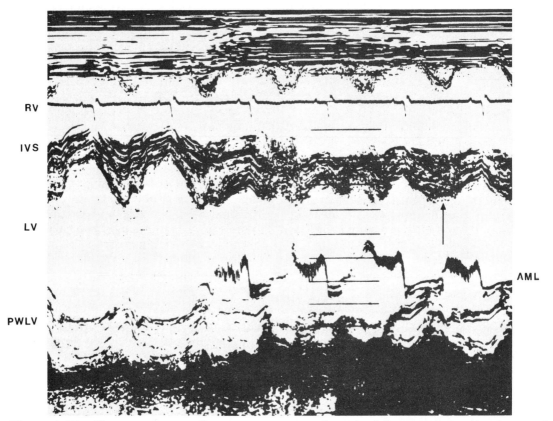

Figure 4–37. Chronic aortic insufficiency. In scanning from the left ventricle (LV) to the mitral valve, the septum (IVS) and the posterior wall of the left ventricle (PWLV) exhibit an exaggerated motion. The E point of the mitral valve is blunted as a result of marked oscillations of the anterior mitral leaflet (AML) throughout diastole. Fine oscillations of the septum are also seen just prior to the mitral E point (arrow) (RV = right ventricle).

Figure 4–38. Oscillations of the anterior mitral leaflet (AML) and the septum (IVS) in chronic aortic insufficiency. Although the diastole opening (E-F) is within normal limits, the amplitude of excursion is reduced to approximately 12 mm. The septal motion is exaggerated, with some septal fluttering prior to the mitral E point. There is marked fluttering of the anterior mitral leaflet throughout diastole.

Figure 4–39. Aortic regurgitation and mitral stenosis. The mitral valve (MV) E-F slope is reduced, with marked leaflet thickening. Upon close observation, fine fluttering is seen in both the septum (IVS) and mitral leaflet throughout diastole (arrow).

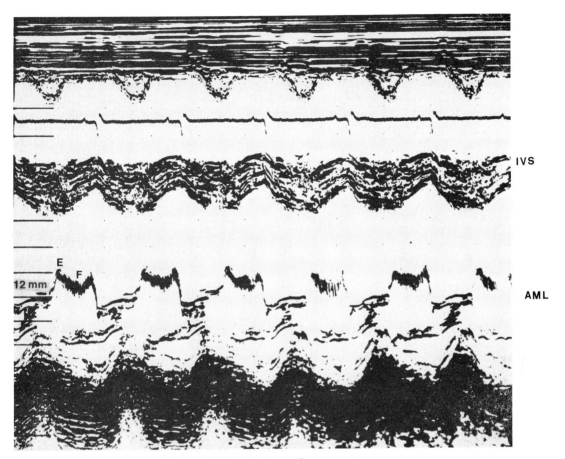

Figure 4–38. See legend on opposite page.

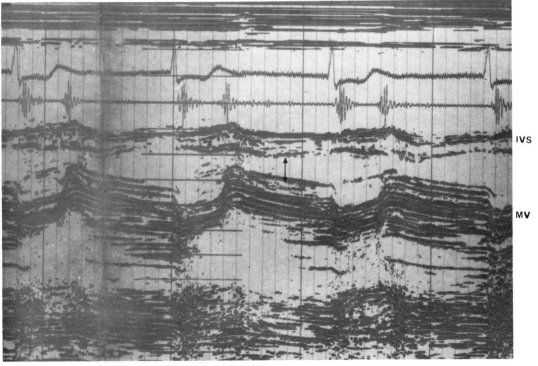

Figure 4–39. See legend on opposite page.

73

nomenon known as the "jet lesion," which consists of an area of fibrosis on either or both of these structures. When the regurgitant flow of aortic insufficiency is intercepted by the septum, as occurred in up to 50 per cent of patients in one series, oscillations similar to those of the mitral valve can be recorded (Fig. 4–37).[60]

The diastolic closure rate (E-F slope) in chronic aortic insufficiency is normal, reduced, or increased.[61] The opening amplitude of the valve (E point) may be reduced (Fig. 4–38). This reduction of the E wave may be caused by the regurgitant flow limiting the valve. When the E-F slope is reduced, mitral scarring due to rheumatic disease (mitral stenosis) is also possible.

In significant aortic insufficiency, the left atrium is usually dilated. When the left atrial dimension exceeds 3.0 cm/per M², however, associated mitral valve disease is usually present.[61a]

In cases of severe mitral stenosis with accompanying aortic insufficiency, the oscillations of the mitral valve may not be seen, owing to the rigidity and thickness of the valve leaflets (Fig. 4–39).

Acute Aortic Insufficiency

There is a definite difference between the echocardiographic appearance of the mitral valve in acute aortic insufficiency and that in chronic aortic insufficiency. In the acute state, the left ventricle is relatively noncompliant. This results in premature diastolic closure of the mitral valve, sometimes resulting in a single opening with the A wave absent. This occurs when the blood enters simultaneously from the left atrium into the left ventricle and from the aorta into the left ventricle through the leaking aortic valve, causing a rapid rise of left ventricular pressure and, therefore, premature closure of the mitral valve (before the beginning of the QRS complex of the electrocardiogram) (Fig. 4–40).[62-66]

The size of the left ventricle is usually normal in early acute aortic insufficiency, but as the disease progresses, the ventricle enlarges. This is to be expected as the ventricle gradually accommodates the extra volume load that is imposed upon it. Additional echocardiographic features include exaggerated posterior wall and septal

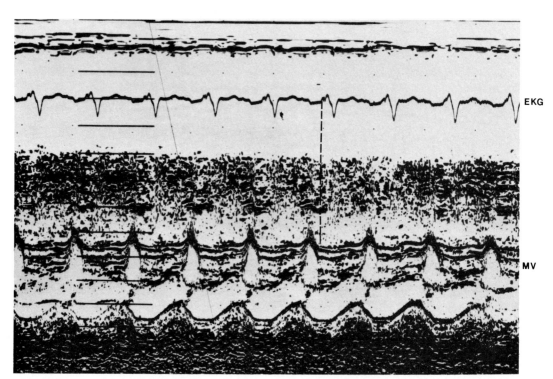

Figure 4–40.   Acute aortic insufficiency in left ventricular failure. The mitral valve (MV) exhibits a single diastolic opening, with marked premature total closure before the onset of the QRS complex. The amplitude of mitral opening is reduced as a result of low flow through the valve in left ventricular failure.

motion as the stroke volume increases (Fig. 4–37).

Thickened Mitral Valve Annulus

The mitral annulus surrounds the mitral orifice and forms the basal attachment of the mitral leaflets.[67] Calcification of the annulus commonly occurs with increasing age.[68] In such patients, calcific deposits frequently coexist on the aortic valve and wall of the aortic root.

The presence of annulus calcification can alter both the function and appearance of the mitral valve. In many cases, it totally obscures the posterior mitral leaflet and appears as an abnormally thickened echo paralleling the posterior aspect of the mitral valve (Fig. 4–41). When performing the echocardiographic recording, caution must be exercised to avoid mistaking the calcified annulus for the posterior left ventricular wall, giving the appearance of a pericardial effusion (Fig. 4–42).

Mitral Stenosis

Mitral stenosis usually occurs as the end result of rheumatic heart disease. In a gradual process, the valve leaflets become fibrotic and thickened and the valve orifice narrows. As the disease progresses, blood flow from the left atrium through the valve becomes impeded. As a result, the left atrial pressure increases, and the left atrial chamber becomes enlarged.

In severe mitral stenosis, it is not uncommon for both leaflets and the chordae tendineae to be involved. This disease is most frequently the result of rheumatic fever and leads to deformity of the mitral valve during the healing process of the disease. Following inflammation of the leaflets and chordae tendineae, there may or may not be deposition of lipids and calcification. The leaflets are thickened and commonly shortened as a result of the chronic scarring process, eventually leading to a total loss of pliability of the leaflets (Fig. 4–43).

In mitral stenosis, the contour of the echocardiographic tracing is significantly altered[9] and produces several classic configurations. In these patients, the diastolic slope of the anterior mitral leaflet, E-F, is reduced to a value that is usually below 35 mm/sec. Other echocardiographic findings include a reduced A wave due to little or no response to atrial systole, and the motion of the posterior leaflet is altered. Normal countermotion of the leaflets in diastole is replaced by a parallel pattern in diastole, a finding in over 90 per cent of cases of mitral stenosis.[69]

Valve mobility may be assessed by measuring the D-E amplitude of excursion, which is usually markedly below the normal range of 20 mm. Reduced mobility is usually seen in the presence of a heavily calcified valve and indicates that the mitral apparatus is also involved in the rheumatic process (Fig. 4–44).[70]

A simultaneous phonocardiogram can be a useful parameter in the assessment of mitral stenosis. With increasing severity of mitral stenosis, the left atrial pressure rises, and as a consequence, the aortic valve closure and mitral valve opening interval, termed the "A_2-OS," shortens (Fig. 4–45).

Alterations in cardiac rhythm, particularly atrial fibrillation, have a profound effect on the diastolic closure rate in patients with mitral stenosis. In these instances, the closure rate should be measured during the longer diastolic periods, as measurements during rapid rates will result in a closure rate disproportionately slowed for the degree of stenosis (Fig. 4–46).

Recording the Stenotic Mitral Valve

As previously emphasized, the key to detecting mitral motion lies in close observation of the A-mode. Compared to the "whiplike" motion of the normal valve on the A-mode, the anterior leaflet of the stenotic valve exhibits a to-and-fro, restricted, rigid type motion. The posterior mitral leaflet also moves with marked restriction. Quite often, the recording between the posterior mitral leaflet and the posterior left ventricular wall appears as a continuous chain of brightly intense echoes.

Final adjustments in instrumentation and angulation should be made from the M-mode prior to actual recording. To avoid false positives or negatives in leaflet thickness, it is necessary to adjust the sensitivity controls, i.e., gain and reject, to where the low-intensity echoes are dampened, but not to the point that the actual thickness of the leaflets cannot be evaluated (Figs. 4–47 to 4–49).

Text continued on page 82

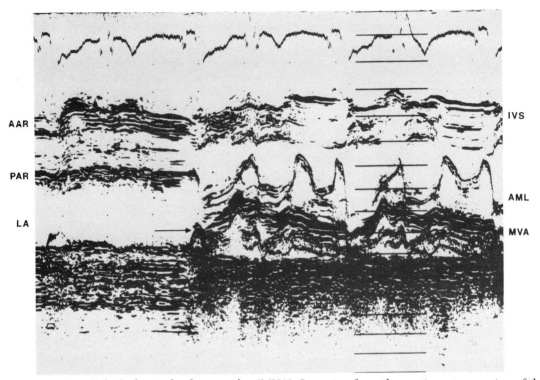

Figure 4-41. Calcified mitral valve annulus (MVA). Scanning from the aortic root, a portion of the calcified mitral annulus is seen protruding into the left atrium (LA) (arrow). The annulus measures approximately 19 mm in thickness (AAR = anterior aortic root; PAR = posterior aortic root; IVS = interventricular septum; AML = anterior mitral leaflet).

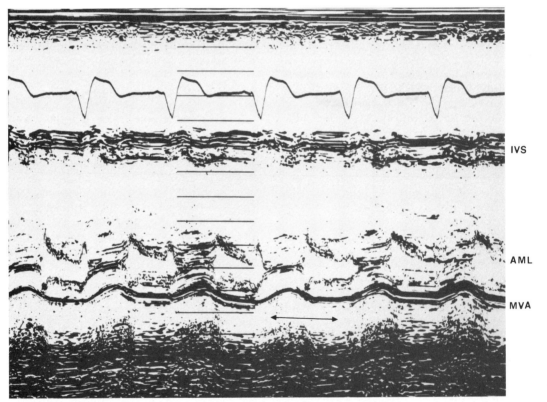

Figure 4-42. Calcified mitral annulus (MVA) simulating pericardial effusion (arrow) (IVS = interventricular septum; AML = anterior mitral leaflet).

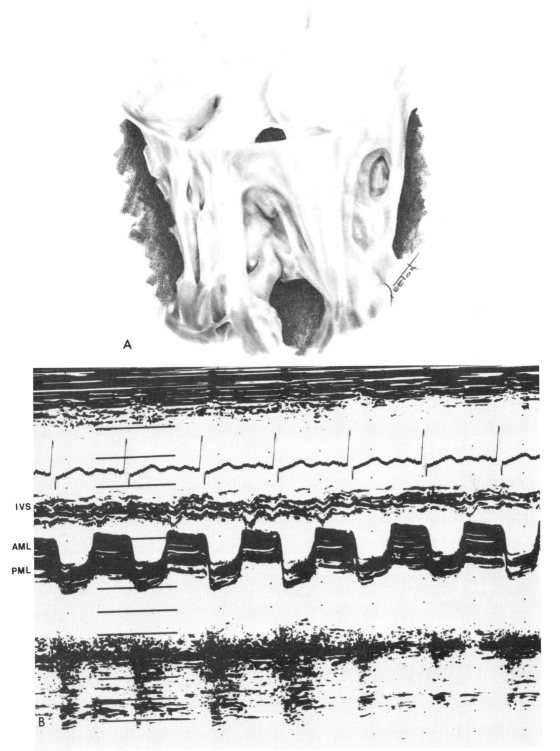

Figure 4-43. (A) Illustration of the scarred mitral valve apparatus of the post-rheumatic type. As compared to Figure 4-2 (the normal mitral apparatus), the components of the stenotic mitral apparatus are thickened and shortened by the fibrotic processes. (B) Echocardiographic recording of severe mitral stenosis. The mitral valve has a box-like appearance with no measurable diastolic closure. The anterior mitral leaflet (AML) is markedly thickened, as is the posterior mitral leaflet (PML) (IVS = interventricular septum).

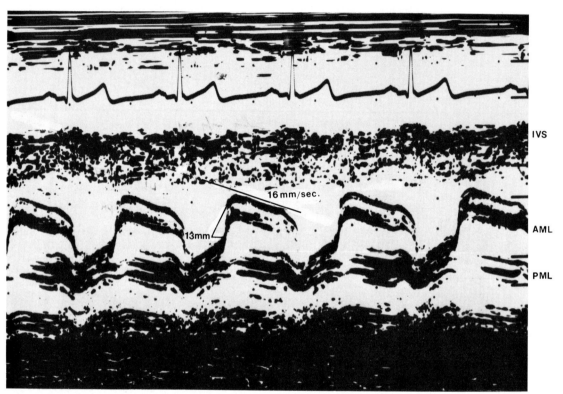

IVS

16 mm/sec.

13mm

AML

PML

Figure 4–44.   Mitral stenosis. The anterior mitral leaflet (AML) is markedly thickened, as is the pos-
terior mitral leaflet (PML), which moves anteriorly with the anterior mitral leaflet during diastole.
The opening amplitude of excursion is reduced to approximately 13 mm. The diastolic descent rate
(E-F) measures approximately 16 mm/sec (IVS = interventricular septum).

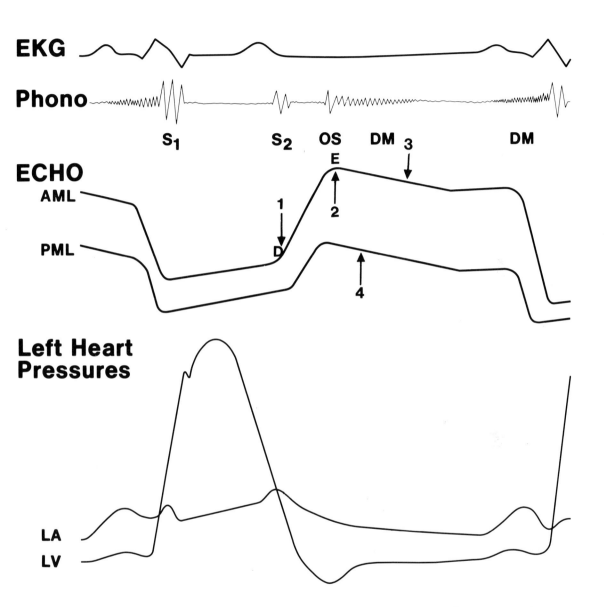

EKG

Phono

S₁   S₂   OS   DM 3   DM

ECHO

AML

PML

Left Heart
Pressures

LA

LV

THE CARDIAC CYCLE: Mitral Stenosis

Figure 4–45. The echocardiographic features of mitral stenosis are illustrated as follows: (1) reduced opening (D-E); (2) rounded E point; (3) slowed diastolic descent slope with an absent F point; and (4) parallel motion of the posterior mitral leaflet (PML) with the anterior mitral leaflet.

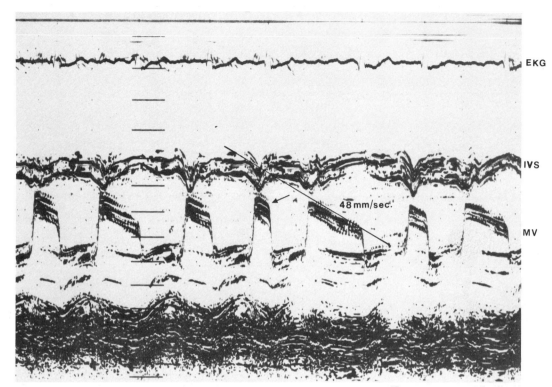

Figure 4-46. Mitral stenosis in atrial fibrillation. The degree of stenosis cannot be evaluated in the presence of a short R-R interval of the electrocardiogram (EKG) (arrow). Only when the rate slows can diastolic closure be measured. Diastolic opening measures approximately 48 mm/sec (IVS = interventricular septum; MV = mitral valve).

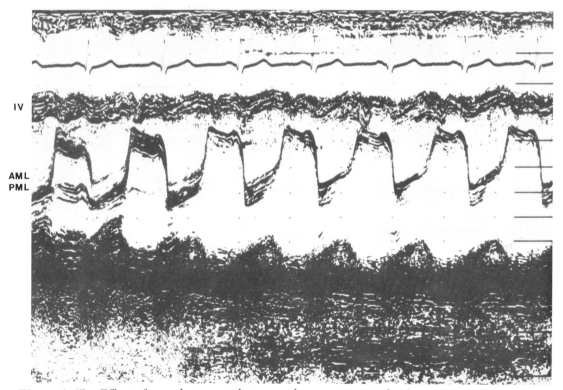

Figure 4-47. Effect of transducer angulation on the stenotic mitral valve. After the first beat, the transducer has been angled slightly superiorly. Compared to the first beat, the following beats show a loss of the posterior mitral leaflet (PML), and the anterior mitral leaflet (AML) loses its thickened appearance. During this period, leaflet thickness cannot be appreciated (IVS = interventricular septum).

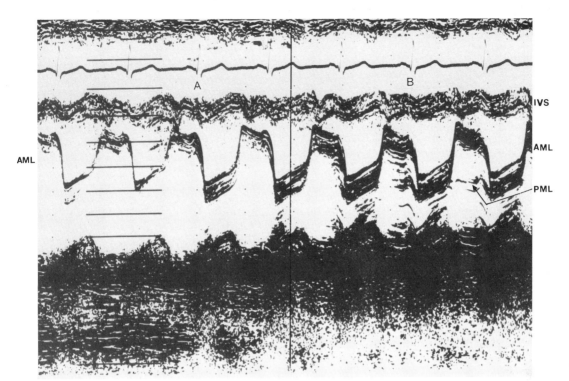

Figure 4–48. Changes in transducer angulation alter the appearance of the stenotic mitral valve. In the section designated A, the anterior mitral leaflet (AML) does not appear thickened in either diastole or systole. The posterior mitral leaflet (PML) is not seen. In the area designated B, the transducer has been directed more inferiorly, and the thickened mitral leaflets are seen throughout the cardiac cycle. The posterior mitral leaflet is seen (arrow) (IVS = interventricular septum).

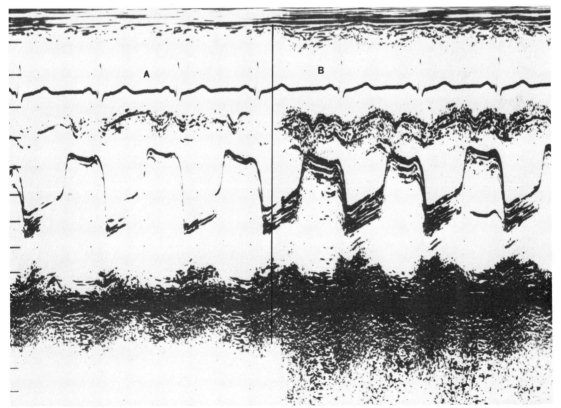

Figure 4–49. Instrumentation settings. In the area designated A, the gain and reject have been improperly adjusted to where the mitral valve echoes cannot be sufficiently viewed. In the area designated B, the error in instrumentation has been corrected, and there is good visualization of the mitral valve.

Mitral Regurgitation

Mitral regurgitation occurs as a result of insufficiency or incompetence of some part of the mitral apparatus, which causes improper closing of the valve. This failure in the leaflets to close properly creates a backflow of blood through the defective valve. Unfortunately, it is not possible by M-mode echocardiography to differentiate between true leaflet separation and multiple beam reflections from various areas of normally functioning mitral leaflets during systole.

Some investigators[71, 72] have found that the increased flow across the valve in mitral incompetence results in an increase in the amplitude or excursion of the valve (D-E) or in an increased rate of closure (E-F).[9] However, in cases in which the valve leaflets are thickened and less pliable, as in combined mitral stenosis and mitral regurgitation, the amplitude and the rate of mitral closure may actually be reduced.[9]

One significant finding that occurs in cases of severe chronic mitral regurgitation is a markedly enlarged left atrium.[71] This, however, would not exclude mitral regurgitation in cases of the acute variety where the atrium has not had time to enlarge to compensate for the increased blood flow. (Figs. 4–29A and 4–50).

Other findings that sometimes occur as a result of mitral regurgitation are (1) an enlarged left ventricle caused by the increased volume of blood being pumped into the chamber; (2) exaggerated septal motion; and (3) a shortening in the duration of the aortic valve opening in systole. This occurs because part of the blood volume that normally would be ejected by the left ventricle through the aortic valve is simultaneously regurgitating back into the left atrium through the insufficient valve. Thus, the left ventricle is not able to maintain its usual pressure throughout systole, and the aortic valve closes prematurely.

Because the above findings are not limited only to mitral regurgitation and because the absence of any of these associated findings does not necessarily exclude the possibility

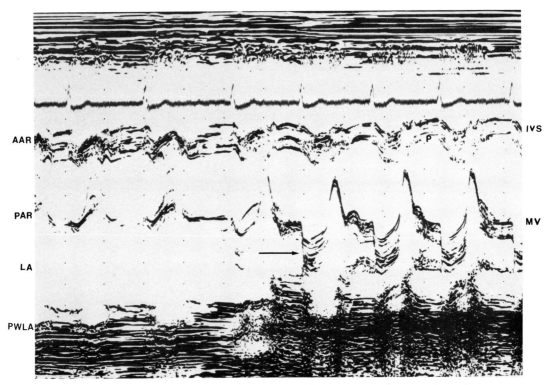

Figure 4–50. Mitral regurgitation secondary to chordal rupture. In this scan from the aortic root to the mitral valve (MV), the position of closure of the mitral valve during systole is displaced in excess of 20 mm behind the posterior wall of the aortic root (PAR) (arrow). The left atrium (LA) is dilated (AAR = anterior aortic root; PWLA = posterior wall of left atrium; IVS = interventricular septum).

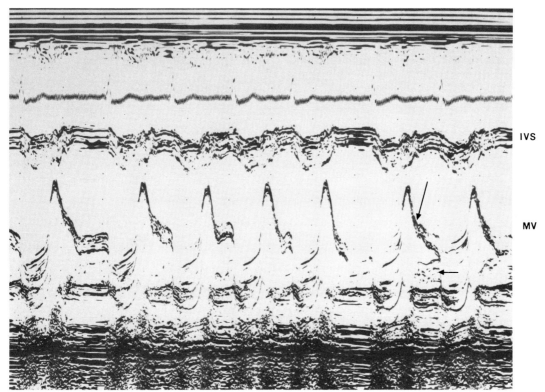

IVS

MV

Figure 4–51. Echocardiogram from a patient with bacterial endocarditis with torn chordae tendineae involving both the anterior and posterior mitral leaflets. Mitral motion is exaggerated. Portions of thickened echoes within the valve presumably originate from vegetations (arrow). During diastole, the anterior leaflet (MV) exhibits coarse fluttering (arrow) (IVS = interventricular septum). Mitral prolapse is evident.

of existing mitral insufficiency, diagnosis of this problem is not possible by means of M-mode echocardiography alone.

Vegetations on the Mitral Valve

In the majority of cases, the formation of mitral leaflet vegetation results from infective endocarditis. Areas of localization of vegetations within the heart are relatively constant, occurring on either the aortic valve or the mitral valve, both of which may be detected echocardiographically.[73] Primary infective endocarditis of the aortic valve frequently causes secondary infection of the mitral valve, the chordae tendineae, and papillary muscles. In this event, the mitral valve cannot seat properly during ventricular systole, and resultant mitral insufficiency may also occur (Fig. 4–51).[74]

Vegetations on the mitral leaflets can usually be characterized by their variable thickness and shaggy appearance (see Figure 4–12). Dillon et al.[73] determined that such vegetations must exceed 2 mm in diameter before they can be detected on the echocardiogram.

REFERENCES

1. Edler I, and Hertz CH: Use of ultrasonic reflectoscope for the continuous recording of movements of heart walls. Kungl Fysiogr Sallsk Lund Forh 24:40, 1954.
2. Friedewald VE Jr. *Textbook of Echocardiography.* Philadelphia, W.B. Saunders Company, 1977.
3. Pohost GM, Dinsmore RE, Rubenstein JJ, O'Keefe DD, Grantham RN, Scully HE, Beierholm EA, Frederiksen JW, Wiesfeldt ML, and Daggett WM: The echocardiogram of the anterior leaflet of the mitral valve: Correlation with hemodynamic and cinero-entgenographic studies in dogs. Circulation 51:88–97, 1975.
4. Rubenstein JJ, Pohost GM, Dinsmore RE, and Harthorne JW: The echocardiographic determination of mitral valve opening and closure: Correlation with hemodynamic studies in man. Circulation 51:98–103, 1975.
5. Shah PM, Gramiak R, Kramer PH, and Yu PN: Determinants of atrial (54) and ventricular (53)

gallop sound in primary myocardial disease. N Engl J Med 278:753, 1968.

6. Edler I, and Gustafson A: Ultrasonic cardiogram in mitral stenosis. Acta Med Scand 195:85, 1957.

7. Joyner CR, Reid JM, Bond JP: Reflected ultrasound in the assessment of mitral valve disease. Circulation 27:503, 1963.

8. Segal BL, Likoff W, and Kingsley B: Echocardiography: Clinical application in mitral stenosis. JAMA 195:161, 1966.

9. Winters WL, Reccetto A, Gimenez J, McDonough M, and Soulen R: Reflected ultrasound as a diagnostic instrument in study of mitral valve disease. Br Heart J 29:788, 1967.

10. Gramiak R, and Shah PM: Cardiac ultrasonography. Radiol Clin North Am 9:469, 1971.

11. Edler I, Gustafson A, Karlefors T, and Christensson B: Ultrasoundcardiography. Acta Med Scand 170(Suppl 370):1, 1961.

12. Gabor GE, and Winsberg F: Motion of mitral valves in cardiac arrythmias (sic): Ultrasonic cardiographic study. Invest Radiol 5:355–360, 1970.

13. Gustafson A, Karlefors T, and Christensson B: Ultrasoundcardiography. Acta Med Scand 170 (Suppl 370):1, 1961.

14. Konecke LL, Feigenbaum H, Chang S, Corya BC, and Fischer JC: Abnormal mitral valve motion in patients with elevated left ventricular diastolic pressures. Circulation 47:989–996, 1973.

15. Borer JS, Henry WL, and Epstein SE: Echocardiographic characteristics of infiltrative cardiomyopathy (Abstr). Circulation (Suppl III) 49, 50:217, 1974.

16. Quiones MA, Gaasch WH, Waisser E, and Alexander JK: Reduction in the rate of diastolic descent of the mitral valve echogram in patients with altered left ventricular diastolic pressure-volume relations. Circulation 49:246–254, 1974.

17. Bass NM, and Sharratt GP: Left atrial myxoma diagnosed by echocardiography, with observations on tumour movement. Br Heart J 35:1332, 1973.

18. Finegan RE, and Harrison DC: Diagnosis of left atrial myxoma by echocardiography. N Engl J Med 282:1022, 1970.

19. Gustafson A, Edler I, Dahlback O, Kaude J, and Persson S: Left atrial myxoma diagnosed by ultrasound cardiography. Angiology 24:554, 1973.

20. Kostis JB, and Moghadam AN: Echocardiographic diagnosis of left atrial myxoma. Chest 58:550, 1970.

21. Schattenberg TT: Echocardiographic diagnosis of left atrial myxoma. Mayo Clin Proc 43:620, 1968.

22. Glasser SP, Bedynek JL, Hall RJ, Hopeman AR, et al.: Left atrial myxoma. Report of a case including hemodynamic, surgical, histologic and histochemical characteristics. Am J Med 50:113–121, 1971.

23. Nasser WK, Davis RH, Dillon JC, et al.: Atrial myxoma: II. Phonocardiographic, echocardiographic, hemodynamic, and angiographic features in nine cases Am Heart J 83:810–824, 1972.

24. Henry WL, Griffith JM, and Epstein SE: Mechanism of left ventricular outflow obstruction in patients with obstructive asymmetric septal hypertrophy (idiopathic hypertrophic subaortic stenosis). Am J Cardiol 35:337–345, 1975.

25. King JF, DeMaria AN, Miller RR, Hilliard GK, Zelis R, and Mason DT: Markedly abnormal mi-tral valve motion without simultaneous intraventricular pressure gradient due to uneven mitral-septal contact in idiopathic hypertrophic subaortic stenosis. Am J Cardiol 34:360–366, 1974.

26. Epstein SE, Henry WL, Clark CE, Roberts WC, Maron BJ, Ferrans VJ, Redwood DR, and Morrow AG: Asymmetric septal hypertrophy. Ann Intern Med 81:650–680, 1974.

27. Abbasi AS, MacAlpin RN, Eber LM, and Pearce ML: Echocardiographic diagnosis of idiopathic hypertrophic cardiomyopathy without obstruction. Circulation 46:897–904, November 1972.

28. Tajik AJ, and Giuliani ER: Echocardiographic observations in idiopathic hypertrophic subaortic stenosis. Mayo Clin Proc 49:89–97, 1974.

29. Popp RL, and Harrison DC: Ultrasound in the diagnosis and evaluation of therapy of idiopathic hypertrophic subaortic stenosis. Circulation 40:905, 1969.

30. Shah PM, Gramiak R, Adelman AG, and Wigle ED: Role of echocardiography in diagnostic and hemodynamic assessment of hypertrophic subaortic stenosis. Circulation 44:891, 1971.

31. Roberts WC, and Cohen LS: Left ventricular papillary muscles: Description of the normal and a survey of conditions causing them to be abnormal. Circulation 46:138–154, 1972.

32. Millward DK, McLaurin LP, and Craige E: Echocardiographic studies of the mitral valve in patients with congestive cardiomyopathy and mitral regurgitation. Am Heart J 85:413–421, 1973.

33. DeBusk RF, and Harrison DC: The clinical spectrum of papillary muscle disease. N Engl J Med 281:1458–1467, 1969.

34. Barlow JB, and Bosman CK: Aneurysmal protrusion of the posterior leaflet of the mitral valve: An auscultatory-echocardiographic syndrome. Am Heart J 71:166–178, 1966.

35. Bittar, M, and Sosa JA: The billowing mitral valve leaflet. Circulation 38:763, 1968.

36. Pomerance A: Ballooning deformity (mucoid degeneration) of atrioventricular valves. Br Heart J 31:343, 1969.

37. Pomerance A: Pathology and valvular heart disease. Br Heart J 34:437–443, 1972.

38. Dillon JC, Haine CL, Chang S, and Feigenbaum H: Use of echocardiography in patients with prolapsed mitral valve. Circulation 49:428, 1974.

39. Gooch AS, Vincenio F, Maranhao V, and Goldberg H: Arrhythmias and left ventricular asynergy in the prolapsing mitral leaflet syndrome. Am J Cardiol 29:611–620, 1972.

40. Pocock WA, and Barlow JB: Postexercise arrhythmias in the billowing posterior mitral leaflet syndrome. Am Heart J 80:740–745, 1970.

41. Goodman D, Kimbiris D, and Linhart JW: Chordae tendineae rupture complicating the systolic click–late systolic murmur syndrome. Am J Cardiol 33:681–684, 1974.

42. Shappell SD, Marshall CE, Brown RE, and Bruce TA: Sudden death and the familial occurrence of mid-systolic click, late systolic murmur syndrome. Circulation 48:1128–1134, 1973.

43. Shappell SD, and Marshall CE: Ballooning posterior leaflet syndrome: Syncope and sudden death. Arch Intern Med 135:664–667, 1975.

44. Weiss AN, Mimbs JW, Ludbrook PA, and Sobel BE: Echocardiographic detection of mitral valve prolapse: Exclusion of false positive diagnosis and

determination of inheritance. Circulation 52:1091–1096, 1975.

45. Sahn DJ, Allen HD, Goldberg SJ, and Friedman WF: Mitral valve prolapse in children. A problem defined by real-time cross-sectional echocardiography. Circulation 53:651, 1976.

46. DeMaria AN, King JF, Bogren HG, Lies JE, and Mason DT: The variable spectrum of echocardiographic manifestations of the mitral valve prolapse syndrome. Circulation 50:33–41, 1974.

47. Popp RL, Brown OR, Silverman JF, and Harrison DC: Echocardiographic abnormalities in the mitral valve prolapse syndrome. Circulation 49:428–433, 1974.

48. Lewis HP: Mid-systolic clicks and coronary heart disease (Editorial). Circulation 44:493–494, 1971.

49. Winkle RA, Goodman DJ, and Popp RL: Simultaneous echocardiographic-phonocardiographic recordings at rest and during amyl nitrite administration in patients with mitral valve prolapse. Circulation 51:522–529, 1975.

50. Fontana ME, Peuce HL, Leighton RF and Wooley CF: The varying clinical spectrum of the systolic click–late systolic murmur syndrome. Circulation 41:807–816, 1970.

51. Sweatman TW, Selzer A, and Cohn K: Echocardiographic diagnosis of ruptured chordae tendineae. Am J Cardiol 26:661, 1970.

52. Duchak JM Jr., Chang S, and Feigenbaum H: Echocardiographic features of torn chordae tendineae. Am J Cardiol 29:260, 1972.

53. Edwards JE: Mitral insufficiency resulting from "overshooting" of leaflets. Circulation 43:606–612, 1971.

54. Selzer A, Kelly JJ Jr., Vannitamby M, Walker P, Gerbode F, and Kerth WJ: The syndrome of mitral insufficiency due to isolated rupture of the chordae tendineae. Am J Med 43:822–836, 1967.

55. Luther RR, and Meyers SN: Acute mitral insufficiency secondary to ruptured chordae tendineae. Arch Intern Med 134:568–578, 1974.

56. Sweatman T, Selzer A, Kamagaki M, and Cohn K: Echocardiographic diagnosis of mitral regurgitation due to ruptured chordae tendineae. Circulation 46:580–586, 1972.

57. Giles TD, Burch GE, and Martinez EC: Value of exploratory "scanning" in the echocardiographic diagnosis of ruptured chordae tendineae. Circulation 49:678–681, 1974.

58. Winsberg F, Gabor GE, Hansberg JG, and Weiss B: Fluttering of the mitral valve in aortic insufficiency. Circulation 41:225, 1970.

59. Edwards JE, and Burchell RB: Endocardial and intimal lesions (jet impact) as possible sites of origin of murmurs. Circulation 18:946–960, 1958.

60. Friedewald VE, Futral JE, Kinard SA, and Phillips B: Oscillations of the interventricular septum in aortic insufficiency (Abstr). In White D (Ed.): Ultrasound in Medicine. New York, Plenum Press, 1975, p. 88.

61. Pridie RB, Benham R, and Oakley CM: Echocardiography of the mitral valve in aortic valve disease. Br Heart J 33:296, 1971.

61a. Unpublished data.

62. Wigle ED, and Labrosse CJ: Sudden, severe aortic insufficiency. Circulation 32:708–720, 1965.

63. Botvinick EH, Schiller NB, Wickramasekaran R, Klausner SC, and Gertz E: Echocardiographic demonstration of early mitral valve closure in severe aortic insufficiency: Its clinical implications. Circulation 51:836–847, 1975.

64. Pridie RB, Benham R, and Oakley CM: Recognition of aortic regurgitation of recent onset by ultrasound technique (Abstr). Am J Cardiol 26:654–655, 1970.

65. Gottlieb S, Khuddus SA, Bolooki H, and Myerburg RJ: Echocardiographic diagnosis of endocarditis (Abstr). Circulation (Suppl III) 49,50:76, 1974.

66. Rees, JR, Epstein EJ, Criley JM, and Ross RS: Haemodynamic effects of severe aortic regurgitation. Br Heart J 26:412–421, 1964.

67. Hirschfeld DS, and Emilson BB: Echocardiogram in calcified mitral annulus. Am J Cardiol 36:354, 1975.

68. Raj MVJ, Bennett DH, Stovin PGI, and Evans DW: Echocardiographic assessment of mitral valve calcification. Br Heart J 38:81, 1976.

69. Abbasi AS, Ellis N, and Child J: Echocardiographic features of infiltrative cardiomyopathy (Abstr). J. Clin Ultrasound 2:221, 1974. (Presented at the Nineteenth Annual Meeting of American Institute of Ultrasound in Medicine, Seattle, Washington, October, 1974.)

70. Gustafson A: Ultrasoundcardiography in mitral stenosis. Acta Med Scand (Suppl) 461:82, 1966.

71. Burgess J, Clark R, Kamigaki M, and Cohn K: Echocardiographic findings in different types of mitral regurgitation. Circulation 48:97–106, 1973.

72. Segal BL, Likoff W, and Kingsley B: Echocardiography: Clinical application in mitral regurgitation. Am J Cardiol 19:50–58, 1967.

73. Dillon JC, Feigenbaum H, Konecke LL, David RH, and Chang S: Echocardiographic manifestations of valvular vegetations. Am Heart J 86:698–704, 1973.

74. Edwards JE: Mitral insufficiency secondary to aortic valvular bacterial endocarditis. Circulation 46:623–626, 1972.

Chapter 5

THE AORTIC ROOT AND THE AORTIC VALVE

Every routine examination includes an adequate recording of the aortic root and the aortic valve. Visualization of the aortic root and aortic valve is important for four reasons: (1) it provides an easily recordable and characteristic landmark in the examination; (2) disease of the aortic valve results in changes in its motion and physical characteristics; (3) the motion of the aortic valve may be altered by changes in left ventricular function; and (4) the aorta itself may be primarily or secondarily altered by disease processes.

ANATOMY

The aortic valve is a semilunar valve, aptly named for its three crescent-shaped cusps. Oxygenated blood is ejected from the left ventricle into the aorta, which is guarded at its entrance by the aortic valve. The strength and relative thickness of this valve are suited to the high pressures to which it is subjected. The three cusps of the valve open into the aortic root lumen during ventricular systole and produce a perfect seal when they close in diastole (Fig. 5–1). The base of each cusp is attached to and suspended from the aortic annulus, with the free, coapting valve edges projecting into the lumen of the vessel. The cusps are of roughly equal size and shape. During ventricular diastole, the cusps fall forcefully into the channel of the vessel, fill with blood, and distend, thereby occluding the vessel to any retrograde flow of blood. It is during this diastolic period that the coronary arteries fill. The aortic root begins at

approximately the third intercostal space. This is also known as the proximal ascending thoracic aorta and is the portion that is recorded by ultrasound.

The aortic valve cusps lie adjacent to the origins of the coronary arteries, hence the nomenclature that designates the two anterior cusps as the right and left coronary cusps. The posterior cusp is also called the noncoronary cusp (Fig. 5–2).

ECHOCARDIOGRAPHIC APPEARANCE

A-Mode Appearance

The echocardiographic identification of the aortic root and aortic valve cusps is primarily dependent upon recognition of the anterior and posterior walls of the aortic root on the A-mode. The appearance of the parallel-moving double echoes of the aortic root is probably the most characteristic of all patterns seen on the echocardiogram. The walls of the aortic root appear as two distinct echo signals of equal amplitude. Moving rapidly between the walls of the aorta, and of lesser amplitude, are the echoes that arise from the aortic valve cusps. Optimally, these cusps are seen as three separate and rather delicate signals (Fig. 5–3).

M-Mode Appearance

On the M-mode display, the echo pattern from the aortic root is very distinctive, comprising two strong echoes that move

Figure 5–1. The aortic valve. In the closed position, the three aortic valve cusps, designated A, B, and C, produce a perfect seal. As shown in this illustration, they are equal in size and circle the inside of the aortic root.

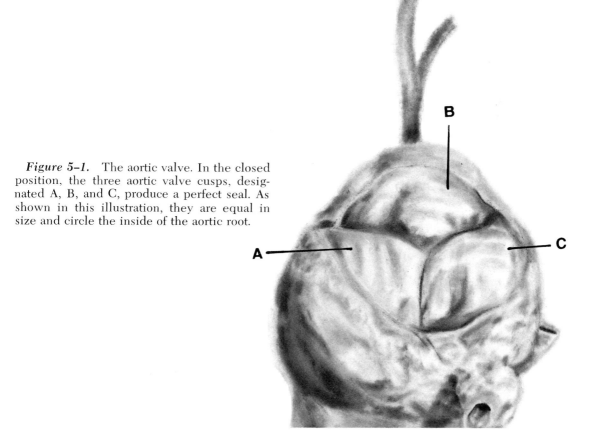

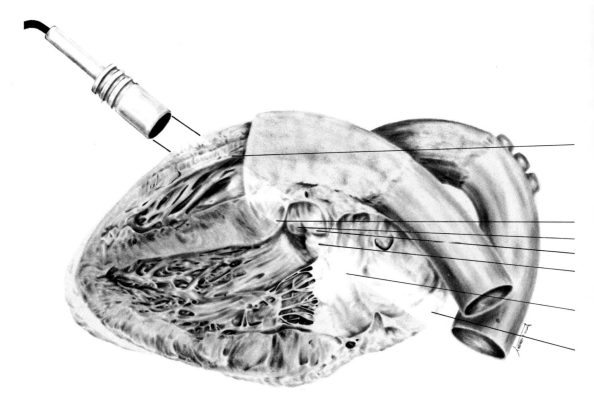

Figure **5–2.** Ultrasound beam through the heart, viewed from the left lateral projection. Key: AWRV = anterior wall of the right ventricle; AAR = anterior aortic root wall; RC = right coronary cusp; LC = left coronary cusp; NC = noncoronary cusp; PAR = posterior aortic root wall; LAC = left atrial chamber; PWLA = posterior wall of the left atrium.

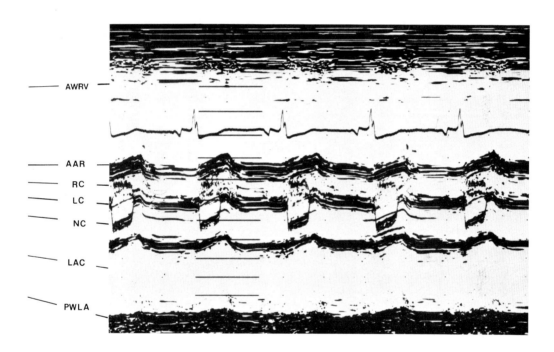

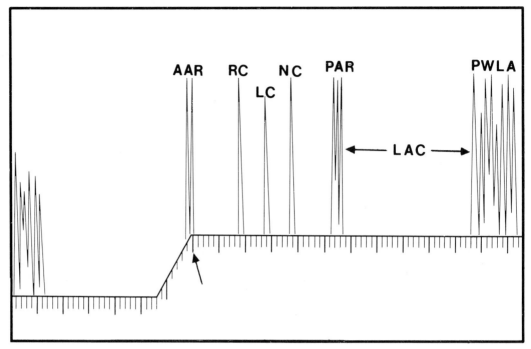

Figure 5–3. A-mode representation of the aortic root and aortic valve. Key: AAR = anterior aortic root wall; RC = right coronary cusp; LC = left coronary cusp; NC = noncoronary cusp; PAR = posterior aortic root wall; LAC = left atrial chamber; PWLA = posterior wall of the left atrium. Note the position of the TGC curve resting against the leading edge of the anterior aortic root wall (arrow).

synchronously about 2.5 to 4.0 cm apart. The anterior echo is reflected from the anterior wall of the aortic root and the posterior echo from the posterior wall of the aortic root. Behind the posterior wall of the aortic root, the left atrial chamber is seen as an echo-free space that is bounded posteriorly by a dense wall of echoes that represent the posterior wall of the left atrium (Fig. 5–2). The motion of the aortic root is the same as that of the other components of the cardiac skeleton, i.e., anterior in direction during ventricular systole and posterior in direction during early diastole.[1] In systole, at the point of the QRS complex of the electrocardiogram, the aortic root begins its anterior excursion that continues until just after the T wave of the electrocardiogram. This motion is then reversed as the aortic root begins to move posteriorly when the pressures in the aorta and left ventricle are equal.[2, 3] At the time of the P wave of the electrocardiogram, the aortic root exhibits a slight posterior motion that coincides with atrial systole before the cycle is then repeated (Fig. 5–4).

In their closed position, during ventricu-lar diastole, the leaflets of the aortic valve form roughly a single plane parallel to the ultrasound beam. The result is a thin band of echoes in approximately the center of the aortic root, with motion that parallels that of the aortic root walls. With the onset of left ventricular systole, the three leaflets part rapidly to form three separate planes as the valve opens.

There is some difference in the nomenclature given to the individual aortic valve cusps. Gramiak and Shah refer to the cusps as the right coronary, the left coronary, and the noncoronary, respectively.[4] Feigenbaum has used the terminology "anterior" (right and left cusps) and "posterior" (noncoronary).[5]

The posterior or noncoronary cusp moves away from the ultrasound transducer into a perpendicular position parallel and adjacent to the posterior wall of the ascending aorta. The right coronary cusp opens anteriorly, and its echo appears adjacent to the anterior aortic wall. The left coronary leaflet usually appears as a slightly off-centered echo between the right coronary and the noncoronary leaflets. This cusp moves later-

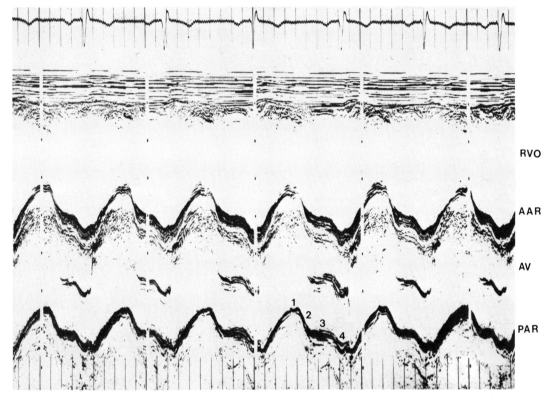

RVO

AAR

AV

PAR

Figure 5-4. Motion of the aortic root. The anterior (AAR) and posterior (PAR) aortic root echoes move in parallel, anteriorly in systole (1) and posteriorly following the completion of ventricular systole (2). The position of the aorta remains relatively fixed during diastole (3) until atrial systole, when an abrupt posterior displacement occurs (4) (RVO = right ventricular outflow tract; AV = aortic valve).

ally in and out of the plane of the ultrasound beam and therefore shows little or no motion and is usually not well recorded.

The opening of the aortic valve occurs when the intraventricular pressure exceeds the aortic pressure. During this period, the aortic root begins its anterior excursion. The cusps close at the end of left ventricular ejection or when the intraventricular pressure falls below the pressure within the aorta (Fig. 5–5). The intervening time, or the duration of aortic valve opening, is the

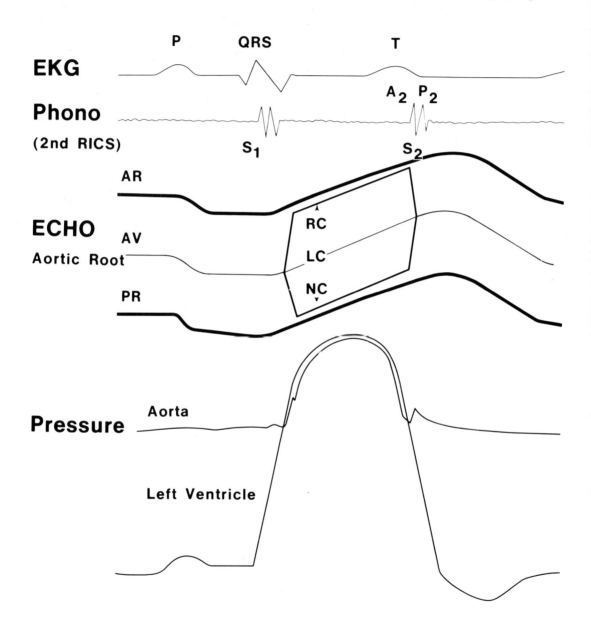

THE NORMAL AORTIC VALVE

Figure 5–5. Schematic illustration of the aortic valve leaflets. Immediately following the QRS complex of the electrocardiogram (EKG), the right coronary (RC), left coronary (LC), and non-coronary (NC) cusps are seen in their open position, forming a "box-like" configuration. Following the T wave of the EKG in diastole, the three leaflets close and form echoes in approximately the center of the aortic root and parallel to the walls of the aortic root. Note that valve opening occurs when the left ventricular pressure exceeds the aortic pressure and closes when the left ventricular pressure falls below the pressure within the aorta.

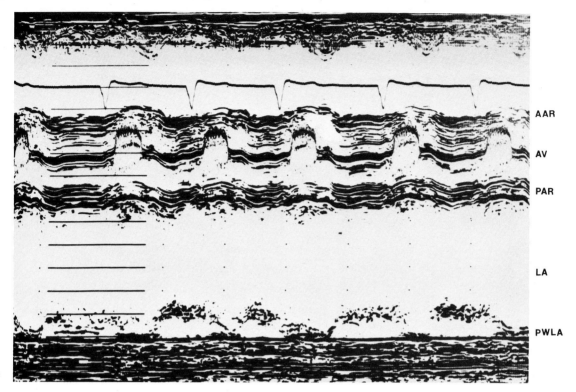

Figure 5-6. Normal, saw-toothed appearance of the aortic valve leaflets. This motion is a normal variant and in this recording is seen best in the right coronary leaflet (arrow). The left atrium (LA) is mildly dilated, and the aortic walls are thickened (AAR = anterior aortic root wall; AV = aortic valve; PAR = posterior aortic root wall; PWLA = posterior wall of the left atrium).

left ventricular ejection time. The ejection time for each cardiac cycle can be determined from the echocardiogram, provided the opening and closing points of the aortic valve leaflets are satisfactorily recorded. During systole, when the aortic valve is open, the separation between the right coronary and noncoronary cusps normally remains constant, or there may be a slight reduction in this dimension from the beginning to the end of systole. During this period, it is not unusual to see the valve cusps exhibit high-frequency vibrations that give them a saw-toothed appearance. These oscillations are presumably caused by the rapid flow of blood across the cusps. Instrumentation and resolution also contribute to the appearance of these fine oscillations (Fig. 5-6). In some cases, the fine systolic oscillations are helpful in distinguishing the aortic valve cusps from the walls of the aortic root.[6]

RECORDING TECHNIQUE

The anatomical relationship of the aortic root to the other cardiac valves makes it a valuable echocardiographic landmark from which these structures may be identified and recorded. Scanning inferiorly and to the left of the aortic root, one moves to the mitral valve, with the anterior wall of the aortic root converging with the interventricular septum (Fig. 5-7). To the right and inferiorly, the anterior wall of the aortic root merges with the membranous septum. Conversely, one may move from the mitral valve to the aortic root.

The mitral valve is the principal echocardiographic landmark in the identification and recording of the aortic root because of its easily recognizable and characteristic M-mode configuration. From the mitral valve position at the third or fourth intercostal space near the sternum, the transducer should be angled medially and superiorly.

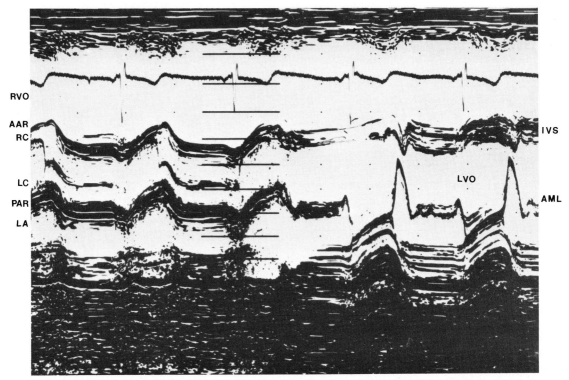

Figure 5–7. Scan from the aortic root to the mitral valve. Directing the transducer slightly inferiorly and laterally from the aortic root, the anterior aortic root (AAR) is continuous with the membranous portion of the interventricular septum (IVS). The posterior aortic root (PAR) is continuous with the anterior leaflet of the mitral valve (AML). The right coronary (RC) and noncoronary (NC) aortic valve leaflets are also recorded. The right ventricular outflow tract (RV) lies anteriorly and the left atrium (LA) posterior to the aortic root (LVO = left ventricular outflow tract).

On the A-mode display, the motion of the anterior mitral leaflet will gradually decrease, and at the same time, the septal echoes will become thinner and move into the motion representative of the aortic root. As the ultrasound beam traverses the aortic root, the echo pattern becomes distinctive, comprising two strong signals that move in unison. The TGC (delay) ramp should be adjusted to rest against the leading edge of the anterior wall of the aortic root. To clarify the echoes, the gain can be adjusted accordingly, and the image can be expanded with the depth control, so that the aortic root, left atrial chamber, and the posterior wall of the left atrium are clearly visualized (Fig. 5–3). Utilization of the A-mode display is of particular importance when looking for the echoes originating from the aortic valve, because the normal aortic valve cusps are thin and open and close extremely rapidly. Once the walls of the aortic root have been locat-

ed, slight angulation of the transducer medially will produce the signals that originate from the aortic valve cusps.

An optimal recording of the aortic valve cusps can demand minute changes in transducer angulation together with slight changes in gain. Even so, because of their anatomical position, it is usually not possible to record all three cusps separately. It is possible, however, to record the right coronary and noncoronary cusps routinely in at least some portion of the cardiac cycle. Simultaneous recording of these two cusps is a good indicator that the correct view of the aortic root and the left atrium is being obtained.

Another indicator of correct transducer placement is the aortic root/left atrial dimension ratio. In the normal subject, the anteroposterior left atrial dimension is approximately the same as the aortic root dimension (Fig. 5–8). Errors in transducer an-

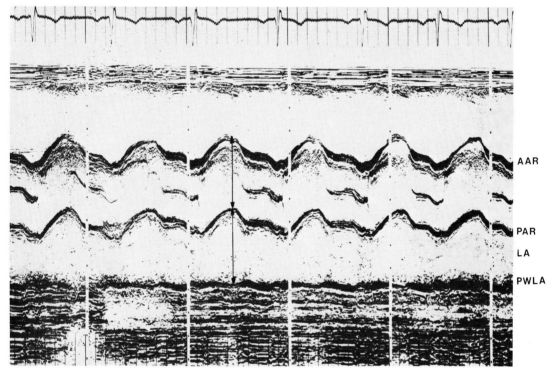

Figure 5–8. In the normal subject, the aortic root and the left atrial dimension (arrows) will be approximately the same (AAR = anterior aortic root; PAR = posterior aortic root; LA = left atrium; PWLA = posterior wall of the left atrium).

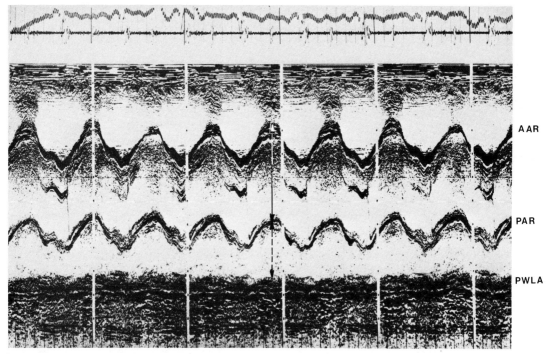

Figure 5-9. With the transducer angled too superiorly, the aortic root dimension is erroneously enlarged and the left atrial dimension reduced. Notice the exaggerated systolic motion of the root (AAR = anterior aortic root; PAR = posterior aortic root; LA = left atrium).

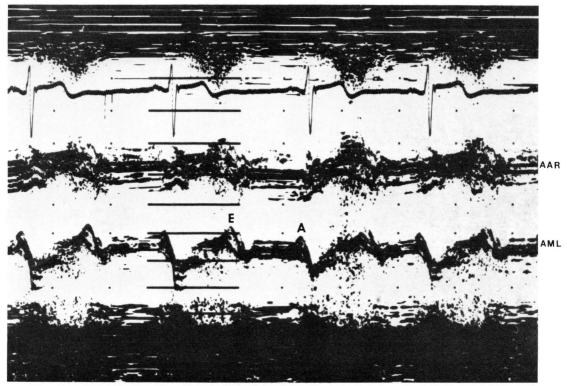

Figure 5–10. Directing the transducer inferiorly when placed too high on the chest. In this recording, the base of the anterior mitral leaflet (AML) may be mistaken for the posterior aortic root wall. The anterior mitral leaflet may be identified by its E and A waves. The excursion of the anterior aortic root is diminished in amplitude, and the edges of the anterior wall are indistinct (AAR = anterior aortic root).

gulation, however, can alter this ratio. When the ultrasound beam transects the aortic root off-center, the recorded dimension can be somewhat smaller than the actual diameter of the structure. This should be considered if the root walls appear unusually thickened. Because the aorta is tubular in configuration, if the beam is oriented too superiorly, more on the long axis of the aorta, exaggerated root motion is displayed, and an erroneously large root dimension will usually be recorded. The left atrium in this case will appear comparatively smaller owing to the ultrasound beam transversing a smaller portion of the atrial cavity (Fig. 5–9). Another error is simulation of the echocardiographic appearance of the aorta by placing the transducer too high and directing the beam inferiorly, so that the anterior aortic wall is recorded together with the base of the anterior mitral leaflet. On such a recording, this part of the anterior mitral leaflet may be mistaken for the posterior aortic wall (Fig. 5–10).

DIMENSION

The Aortic Root

Aortic root measurements are made at the beginning of the QRS complex of the electrocardiogram in the section of the aorta in which there is simultaneous visualization of the aortic valve cusps. It is at this time that the measurements are the most reproducible. At the present time, the method of measuring the aortic root dimension varies among different laboratories. The method that is probably used most often involves measuring the distance between the anterior edge of the anterior wall of the aortic root and the edge of the posterior wall of the aortic root. A second and probably better method of measuring the dimension of the aortic root is to measure the distance between the anterior edges of both the anterior and posterior walls of the aortic root, leading edge to leading edge (Fig. 5–11). In adults, the normal dimension of the aortic

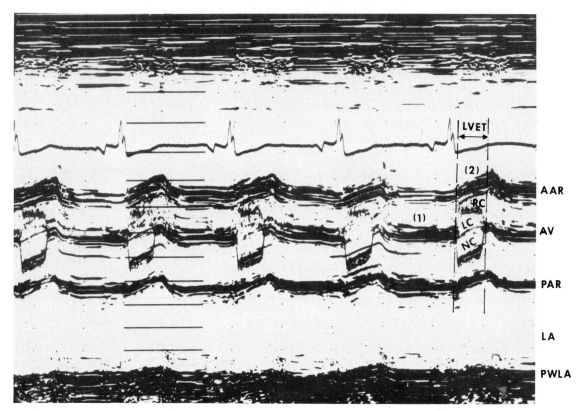

Figure. 5-11. In diastole (1), between the T wave and the QRS complex of the electrocardiogram, the aortic valve (AV) is in its closed position. In this position it is recognized as a single band of echoes within the center of the aortic root. In systole (2), following the QRS complex of the electrocardiogram, the aortic valve opens, creating a "box-like" configuration. From anterior to posterior are the right coronary (RC), left coronary (LC), and noncoronary (NC) cusps. The aortic valve orifice dimension is measured from the right coronary cusp to the noncoronary cusp. The left ventricular ejection time (LVET) is the duration of actual ejection from the left ventricle (AAR = anterior aortic root; PAR = posterior aortic root; LA = left atrium; PWLA = posterior wall of left atrium).

root varies between 2.0 and 3.8 cm,[1, 4] most frequently averaging between 2.5 and 3.5 cm.

The Aortic Valve

During systole, when the aortic valve is in a fully open position, the separation between the right coronary and the noncoronary leaflets remains relatively constant. In adults, the distance from the right coronary cusp to the noncoronary cusp is normally about 2.0 cm, with a normal range of 1.7 to 2.5 cm (Fig. 5–11).

In the normal heart, the duration of aortic valve opening, or the left ventricular ejection time, is principally a function of the heart rate. Patients with varying R-R intervals, such as in atrial fibrillation and premature ventricular contractions, will show corresponding variations in the left ventricular ejection time, with a longer duration of ejection after longer diastolic filling periods. During a premature ventricular contraction, the aortic valve may fail to open at all, or, more frequently, it will exhibit only an abbreviated opening. The first beat after the premature ventricular contraction will then show a longer ejection time (Fig. 5–12).

ALTERATIONS OF THE AORTIC VALVE AND AORTIC ROOT

Aortic Stenosis

Aortic stenosis is obstruction of the outflow tract of the left ventricle above (supravalvular stenosis), below (subvalvular

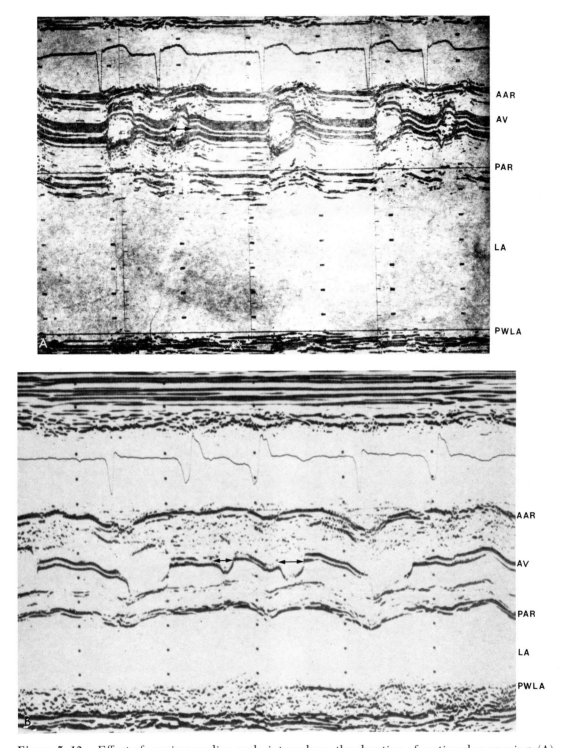

Figure 5-12. Effect of varying cardiac cycle intervals on the duration of aortic valve opening. (A) Atrial fibrillation. The aortic valve opening time is directly proportional to the duration of the previous diastolic period (arrows). (B) Premature ventricular contractions (PVCs). The first and fourth beats have normal aortic valve opening. The second and third beats are PVCs with markedly abbreviated duration of valve opening (arrows) (AAR = anterior aortic root; AV = aortic valve; PAR = posterior aortic root; LA = left atrium; PWLA = posterior wall of left atrium).

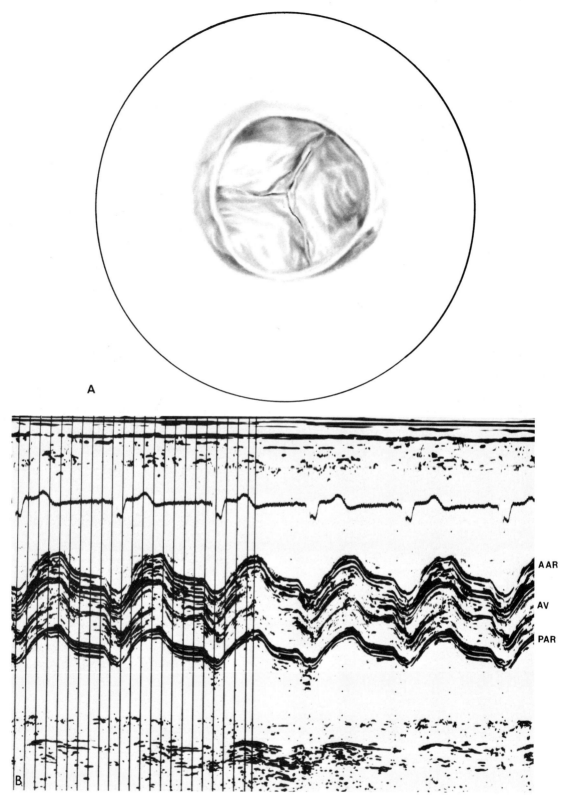

Figure 5–13. (A) The diseased aortic valve. The aortic cusps are thickened, preventing normal functioning of the valve apparatus. Note that the cusps at the point of closure are irregular and are not able to seal properly. (B) Aortic stenosis. The diastolic leaflet echoes are increased, and the leaflet separation in systole is restricted (AAR = anterior aortic root; AV = aortic valve; PAR = posterior aortic root).

stenosis), or at the level of the aortic valve (valvular stenosis). Valvular stenosis may be caused by calcification and sclerosis of a congenitally deformed valve, or it may occur secondarily to rheumatic valvulitis.

In most cases of aortic stenosis, the cusps of the aortic valve are thick, rigid, and markedly distorted in appearance. Vegetations deposited across the surface of the valve lead to scarring and fusion of the individual cusps. The echoes arising from this area are markedly thickened. The walls of the aortic root frequently exhibit a rigid motion instead of the free, undulating, parallel motion characteristic of the normal aortic root. The density of the echoes from the region of the aortic valve generally, but not invariably, increases in proportion to the degree of obstruction (Fig. 5–13). These abnormal echoes are caused by calcification and fibrosis of the valve leaflets and annulus.

The normal aortic valve reflects three or fewer echoes in diastole that are lighter in intensity than those of the walls of the aorta.[4] In mild aortic stenosis, the number of diastolic echoes is increased, with slight restriction of the valve (Fig. 5–14), and the valve leaflets lose their thin, attenuated appearance, particularly if calcium is present. As the severity of stenosis increases, the echoes within the aortic root increase in density until the entire aortic root is filled with an almost continuous band of echoes paralleling the normal movements of the aorta (Fig. 5–15). Aortic valve disease with no mitral disease is usually a congenital problem rather than rheumatic valvulitis. Conversely, combined aortic and mitral disease is almost always rheumatic (Fig. 5–16).

A good ultrasonic recording of the leaflets themselves in aortic stenosis is often difficult to obtain, and the echocardiographic estimation of aortic stenosis is hazardous even under the best circumstances. This is

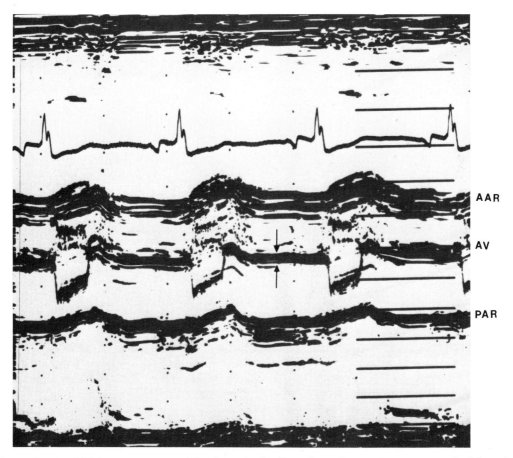

Figure 5–14.   Mild aortic stenosis. The diastolic leaflet echoes (arrows) are increased, although the leaflet separation in systole appears preserved. The systolic echoes are also thickened (AAR = anterior aortic root; AV = aortic valve; PAR = posterior aortic root).

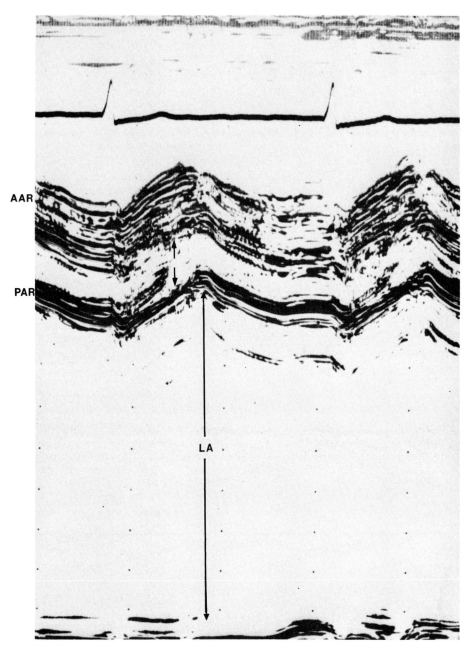

Figure 5–15. Severe aortic stenosis. The entire aortic root appears as a mass of dense echoes, with only faintly discernible valvular systolic opening and closure (arrows). There is severe left atrial enlargement (LA) (AAR = anterior aortic root; PAR = posterior aortic root).

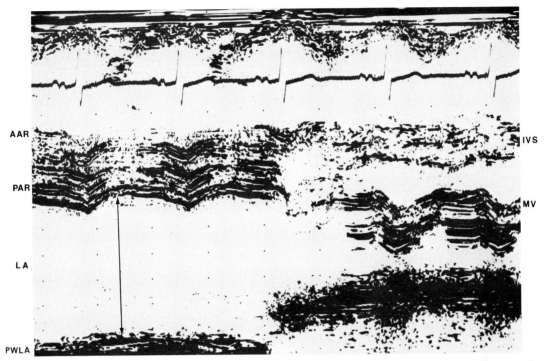

Figure 5-16. Concomitant rheumatic aortic stenosis and mitral stenosis. Discrete aortic valve leaflet motion is not discernible as the aortic root is filled with echoes due to scarring of the valve. The mitral valve (MV) is markedly thickened, with a flattened E-F slope. The left atrium (LA) is dilated (arrow) (AAR = anterior aortic root; PAR = posterior aortic root; PWLA = posterior wall of the left atrium; IVS = interventricular septum).

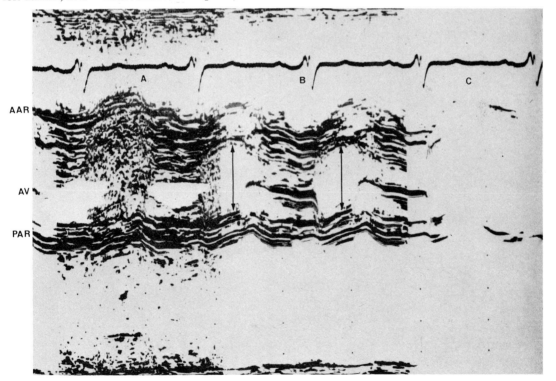

Figure 5-17. Gain adjustment in severe aortic stenosis. Plane A shows use of excessively low gain setting, resulting in excessive echoes that obscure leaflet separation. Plane B demonstrates correct use of the gain, with discernible leaflet separation in systole (arrows). In plane C, the echoes are virtually erased owing to overuse of both the gain and reject (AAR = anterior aortic root; AV = aortic valve; PAR = posterior aortic root).

103

particularly true in those subjects with calcific aortic stenosis where thick, multi-layered complexes are seen within the confines of the aortic root and the usual aortic valve cusp architecture is lost. The most reliable method of evaluating aortic stenosis is to first identify the aortic root on the A-mode display. The gain should then be adjusted to visualize the walls of the aorta and the aortic valve cusps. A small amount of reject is often helpful in eliminating those echoes that originate from the calcific areas. Overzealous use of the gain and reject, however, can make the degree of stenosis appear either more or less severe than it actually is (Fig. 5-17). It should be emphasized that even with optimal recordings, in most cases of aortic stenosis, the disease process obliterates the usual landmarks, making measurement of valvular motion difficult or impossible.

Idiopathic Hypertrophic Subaortic Stenosis (IHSS)

A definite alteration of aortic valve motion may be seen in many subjects with IHSS.[7] Although the aortic valve opens normally, it often partially closes in mid-systole, then

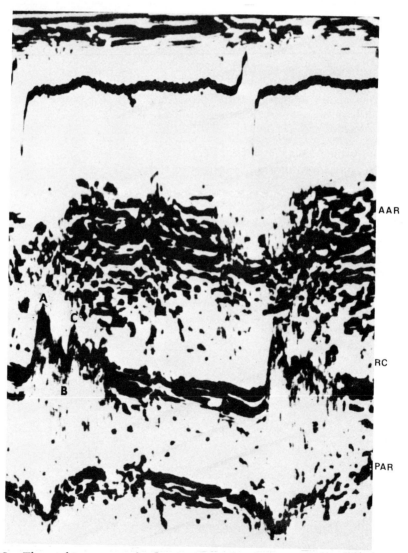

Figure 5–18. The right coronary leaflet in idiopathic hypertrophic subaortic stenosis (IHSS). Following early systolic opening (A), the valve partially closes in mid-systole (B), and reopens in late systole (C) (RVO = right ventricular outflow tract; AAR = anterior aortic root; RC = right coronary cusp; PAR = posterior aortic root).

reopens late in systole. Coarse systolic fluttering of the aortic leaflets may be more marked than is normally seen (Fig. 5–18).[8]

Discrete Subaortic Stenosis

The characteristic, although not diagnostic, echocardiographic findings in those patients with discrete membranous subaortic stenosis are as follows:

1. Rapid opening of the aortic valve leaflets with the onset of systole followed by an abrupt closure.[9, 11, 12]
2. The valve remains partially closed throughout the remainder of systole.
3. The valve leaflets frequently exhibit a gross fluttering throughout the remainder of systole, possibly caused by a jet-stream effect of the turbulent blood flow striking the leaflets.[11]
4. An absence of the characteristic systolic anterior motion (SAM) of the mitral valve observed in idiopathic hypertrophic subaortic stenosis.[2, 11]

The premature closure of the valve is believed to be caused by obstruction of aortic valve flow produced by a ring-like fibrous band of tissue usually located immediately below the aortic valve. (The premature aortic valve closure is similar to a pattern frequently seen in obstructive asymmetric septal hypertrophy, although with that condition, the leaflets characteristically completely reopen in mid- to late systole.[2] In a variation of this abnormal valve motion, there is normal initial separation of the leaflets, but before the full open position is reached, the opening rate slows.[10])

The rapid jet of blood onto the aortic valve leaflets subjects them to trauma that may result in leaflet deformity with calcification and fibrosis (Fig. 5–19).[2, 13]

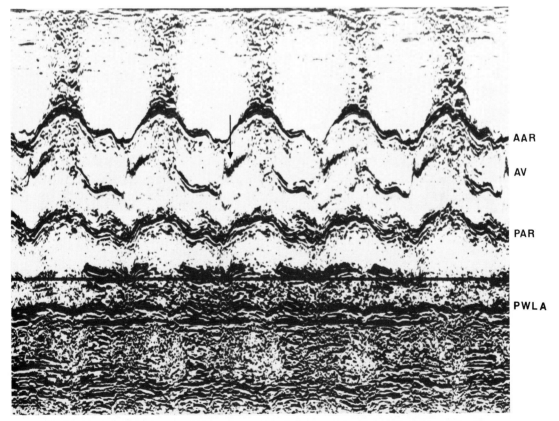

Figure 5–19. Aortic valve motion in discrete subaortic stenosis. Normal initial leaflet opening is followed by premature partial closure (arrow) for the duration of ventricular systole (AAR = anterior aortic root; AV = aortic valve; PAR = posterior aortic root; PWLA = posterior wall of left atrium).

Aortic Regurgitation

The echocardiographic signs of both chronic and acute aortic regurgitation are best seen in the following abnormalities in the appearance of cardiac structures:

1. Repetitive oscillations of the anterior, and less often, posterior, mitral valve leaflets during diastole.[14, 15] This is particularly true in those patients with isolated chronic aortic insufficiency. In some cases with associated mitral stenosis, the diastolic fluttering of the mitral valve is not seen, probably because of the loss of leaflet pliability. Diastolic fluttering of the mitral valve is produced by the regurgitant flow of blood through an incompetent aortic valve as it strikes the anterior mitral leaflet (Fig. 5–20).[16] There is no correlation between the presence or severity of the oscillations and the severity of the regurgitation.[17]

2. The amplitude of excursion is reduced, and the E point of the mitral valve is usually flattened, primarily because the regurgitant flow limits the valve opening (Fig. 5–21). When mitral opening is abbreviated

in these cases, the E-F slope is not a valid measurement as a reflection of flow rate across the valve and therefore should not be measured.

3. True premature closure of the mitral valve is a hallmark of acute severe aortic regurgitation (although it is also seen in first degree heart block). Because the left ventricle is small and unable to distend rapidly enough, the left ventricular pressure quickly exceeds the left atrial pressure and abruptly closes the mitral valve soon after it has opened (Fig. 5–22).

4. Diastolic fluttering and exaggerated motion of the interventricular septum. When the regurgitant flow of aortic insufficiency is intercepted by the septum, oscillations similar to those of the mitral valve can be recorded (Fig. 5–23).[18] In those cases of mitral stenosis, septal oscillations are helpful in determining the presence of associated aortic insufficiency. Similar oscillations are less frequently observed on the chordal echoes and from the posterior left ventricular endocardial surface.

5. Dilatation of the left ventricle. In chronic regurgitation, the increased volume imposed on the left ventricle is manifested

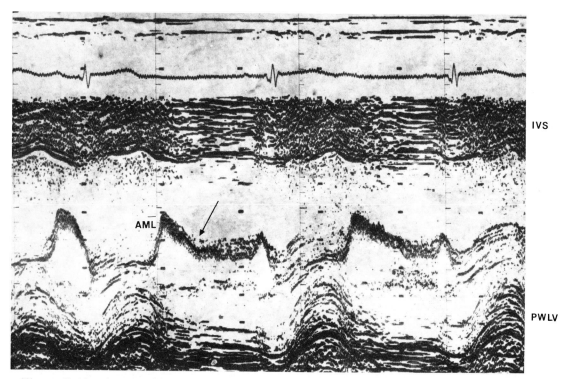

Figure 5–20. Aortic regurgitation. The anterior mitral leaflet (arrow) exhibits fine oscillations. The interventricular septum (IVS) is hypertrophied (PWLV = posterior wall of the left ventricle).

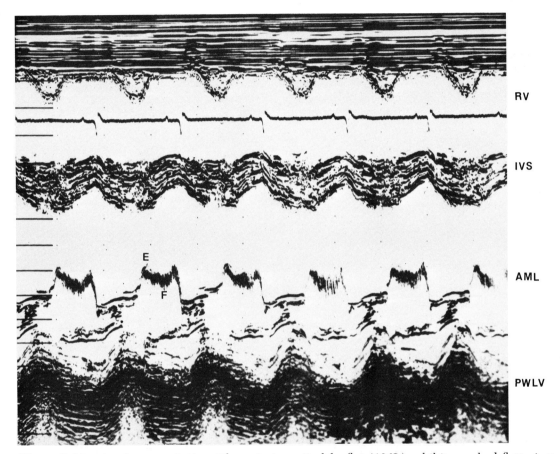

RV

IVS

AML

PWLV

Figure 5–21. Aortic regurgitation. The anterior mitral leaflet (AML) exhibits marked fluttering, and the E point is slightly blunted, with a reduced E-F slope. The marked fluttering of the anterior mitral leaflet prevents measurement of the E-F slope. The interventricular septum (IVS) exhibits exaggerated systolic motion (RV = right ventricle; PWLV = posterior wall of the left ventricle).

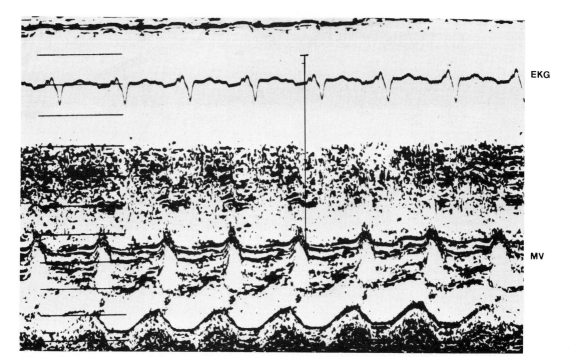

Figure 5-22. Acute aortic regurgitation. The mitral valve (MV) exhibits a single diastolic opening, with marked premature total closure before the onset of the QRS complex of the electrocardiogram (EKG) (arrow).

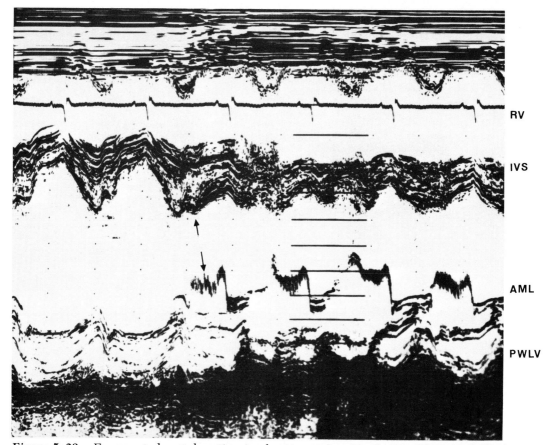

Figure 5-23. Exaggerated septal motion in chronic aortic regurgitation. The septal (IVS) motion is exaggerated, with marked fluttering of both the septum and the anterior mitral leaflet (AML) (arrows). Notice how the hyperdynamic motion of the septum is more apparent below the level of the mitral valve (RV = right ventricle; PWLV = posterior wall of the left ventricle).

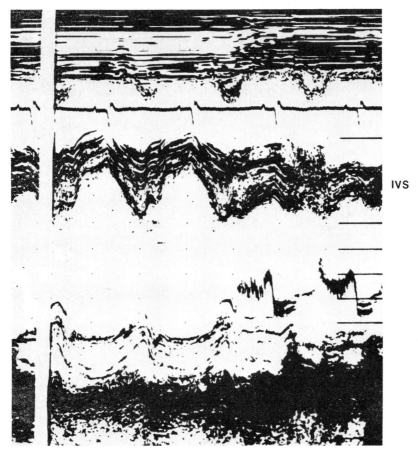

IVS

Figure 5-24. Exaggerated septal (IVS) motion, in aortic regurgitation. The large end-diastolic dimension results in an ejection fraction of approximately 42 per cent.

by dilatation of that chamber many years before actual left ventricular failure occurs. The posterior wall exhibits an exaggerated motion. This hyperdynamic left ventricular wall motion results in a disproportionately large end-diastolic dimension compared to the end-systolic dimension, a manifestation of an increased ejection fraction (Fig. 5–24).

Acute aortic regurgitation may occur after perforation of a cusp in infective endocarditis or after sudden expansion of the aortic root in dissecting aneurysms. Regardless of cause, acute aortic regurgitation is frequently a genuine medical emergency in which cardiac catheterization may not be feasible. The important difference between acute and chronic aortic insufficiency is the ability of the left ventricle to accommodate the slowly progressive chronic form and its relative inability to adjust to the acute volume overload.[2, 19, 20] Hemodynamically, in acute aortic insufficiency, there is a rapid balance of the aortic and left ventricular pressures. As seen in Figure 5–22, the mi-

tral valve closes before the onset of the QRS complex. Other features include delayed diastolic opening and curtailment of diastolic mitral valve opening amplitude. These echocardiographic features can be helpful in diagnosing acute aortic insufficiency and thus circumvent catheterization prior to aortic valve replacement.

The echocardiographic appearance of the aortic valve and aortic root are usually abnormal in aortic regurgitation, but the exact findings depend on the underlying cause: Incompetency of the aortic valve may be due to disease of the valve tissue itself or may result from dilatation of the aortic root. The aortic valve leaflets are sometimes difficult to record in aortic insufficiency (Fig. 5–25).[2]

In aortic regurgitation, irrespective of the cause, the aortic root is usually dilated or is at least at the upper limits of normal width. Together with dilatation of the aortic root in fully compensated aortic regurgitation, the aortic valve sometimes exhibits an increased duration of opening; hence, the left ventricular ejection time may be prolonged.[2] This

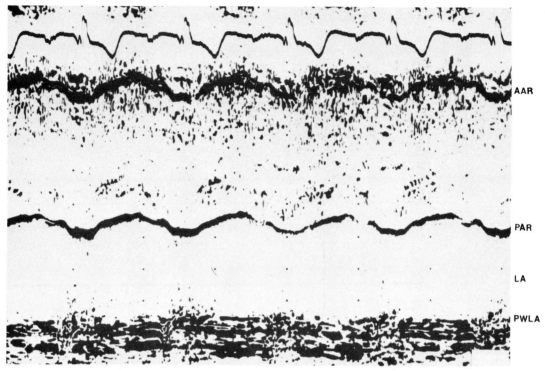

AAR

PAR

LA

PWLA

Figure 5-25.   Chronic aortic regurgitation. The aortic root is dilated in comparison to the left atrium (LA), and the aortic root appears "empty," with poor definition of leaflet echoes (AAR = anterior aortic root; PAR = posterior aortic root; PWLA = posterior wall of the left atrium).

may not be apparent, however, unless the leaflets are not thickened and are well recorded.

It must be emphasized that although patients with aortic regurgitation show a slightly wider root and some related increase in systolic cusp movement, these findings alone do not present an ultrasonic pattern that is diagnostic of aortic regurgitation.

THE AORTIC VALVE AND CARDIAC OUTPUT

The duration of aortic valve opening and aortic valve motion reflect the flow across the valve. The size of the valve orifice, the velocity of flow, and the left ventricular ejection time are all functions of aortic flow. There are a number of clinical instances in which the aortic valve cusp movements are influenced by reduced flow across the aortic valve. Some of these include (1) varying R-R intervals, such as occur in atrial fibrillation where both the orifice dimension and left

ventricular ejection time vary from beat to beat; and (2) during a premature ventricular contraction, the aortic valve may fail to open at all, or more frequently, it will exhibit only abbreviated opening. The first beat after the premature ventricular contraction will then show a longer ejection time (Fig. 5-12B). Other clinical instances that produce a reduced flow across the aortic valve include mitral stenosis (Fig. 5-26), left ventricular dysfunction, such as coronary artery disease (Figs. 5-27 and 5-28), and mitral regurgitation.

CALCIFICATION OF THE AORTIC ROOT

It is a common echocardiographic finding to see calcification of the aortic root walls in elderly patients. An associated finding in these cases is frequently the presence of a calcified mitral annulus.[2] Transducer angulation can produce false thickening of the aortic root walls, especially if the ultrasound beam strikes the aortic root in an oblique

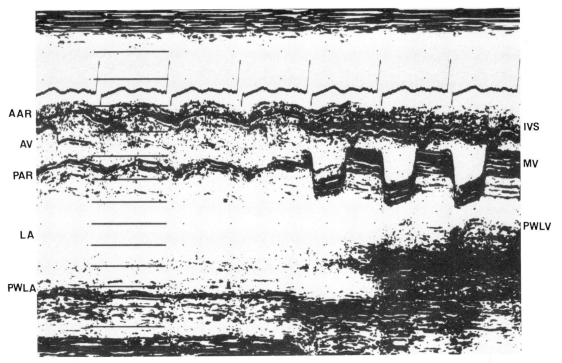

Figure 5-26. Reduced opening of a normal aortic valve in mitral stenosis. On this sweep from the aortic valve (AV) to the highly stenotic mitral valve (MV), the aortic valve exhibits a reduced opening. It does, however, appear pliable. The left atrium (LA) is markedly dilated (AAR = anterior aortic root; PAR = posterior aortic root; PWLA = posterior wall of the left atrium; IVS = interventricular septum; PWLV = posterior wall of the left ventricle).

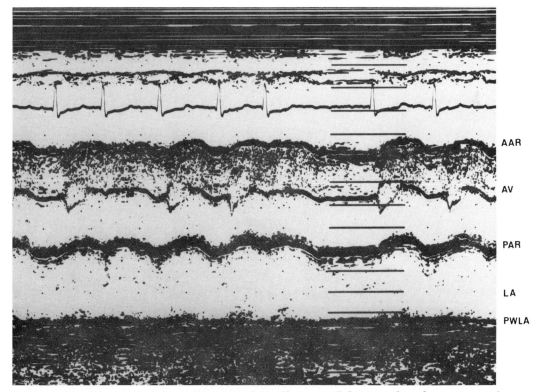

Figure 5-27. The aortic valve (AV) in atrial fibrillation and decreased cardiac output. There is a markedly decreased opening of the aortic valve due to a low cardiac output and left ventricular failure. Following the second and fifth beats, there is no apparent valve opening (AAR = anterior aortic root; PAR = posterior aortic root; LA = left atrium; PWLA = posterior wall of the left atrium).

111

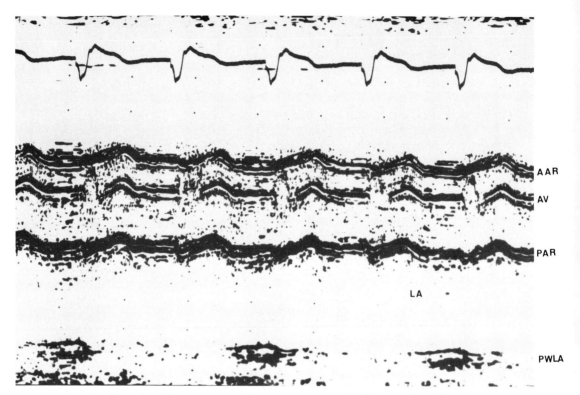

AAR

AV

PAR

LA

PWLA

Figure 5–28. Patient with severe mitral regurgitation with decreased cardiac output. The aortic valve (AV) appears small within the center of the aorta (AAR = anterior aortic root; PAR = posterior aortic root; LA = left atrium; PWLA = posterior wall of left atrium).

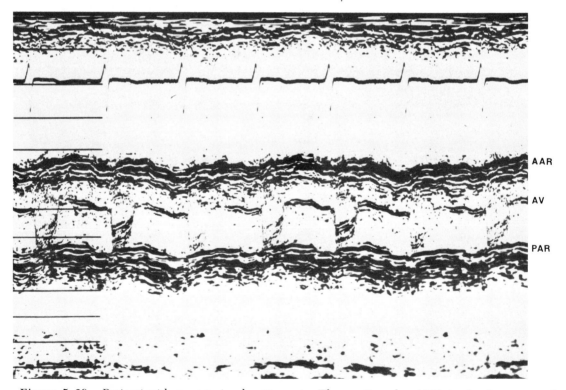

AAR

AV

PAR

Figure 5–29. Patient with an arteriosclerotic aorta. The aortic valve (AV) is clearly seen and appears pliable within the thickened walls of the aorta (AAR = anterior aortic root; PAR = posterior aortic root).

112

manner. However, when the aortic valve leaflets are clearly seen within the walls of the aorta, one can be reasonably sure that calcification of the aortic root walls does exist when the walls are thick (Fig. 5–29).

On the A-mode display, the walls of the aorta will appear as two signals of much brighter intensity than the normal aortic root signals.

THE PHONOCARDIOGRAM IN AORTIC VALVE DISEASE

The phonocardiogram is not essential in evaluating aortic valve disease, but it may be of interest to the physician when used simultaneously with the echocardiographic recording. Aortic valve murmurs are best heard along the left sternal border and second right intercostal space. Placement of the phonocardiographic transducer in either the second or third intercostal space, close to the sternum, will usually provide maximum identification of the aortic valve mur-mur. The murmurs of aortic stenosis and aortic regurgitation in some instances can be identified by placing the phonocardiographic transducer at the second or third intercostal space along the right sternal border. Both positions, right and left, should be attempted to obtain the best phonocardiographic recording.

TECHNICAL ERRORS

In addition to the technical errors previously discussed in this chapter, other commonly recorded errors and methods that can be employed to correct them are illustrated in Figures 5–30 to 5–34.

AORTIC VALVE VEGETATIONS

Dense thickenings of the normally thin aortic cusps are highly suggestive of infective vegetations.[21-23] The presence of vegetations should especially be suspected

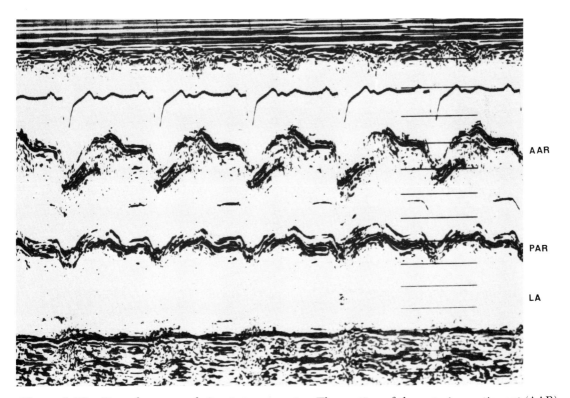

Figure 5–30. Transducer angulation is too superior. The motion of the anterior aortic root (AAR) appears exaggerated, while the motion of the posterior aortic root (PAR) is diminished and reduced in amplitude. The aortic root dimension is greater than that of the left atrium (LA).

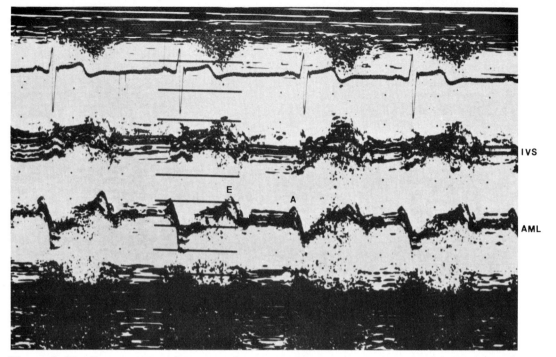

Figure 5–31. Incorrect transducer angulation. In this view, the ultrasonic beam is striking the area just inferior to the aortic root, producing an echocardiographic configuration that closely simulates the echoes of the anterior and posterior aortic root walls. The beam, however, is actually striking the upper portions of the interventricular septum (IVS) and the anterior mitral valve leaflet (AML). This is further confirmed by its M-shaped configuration and the distinct presence of an E point. In this view, neither the mitral valve, aortic root, nor left atrium can be accurately measured. Note also the presence of a mitral A wave.

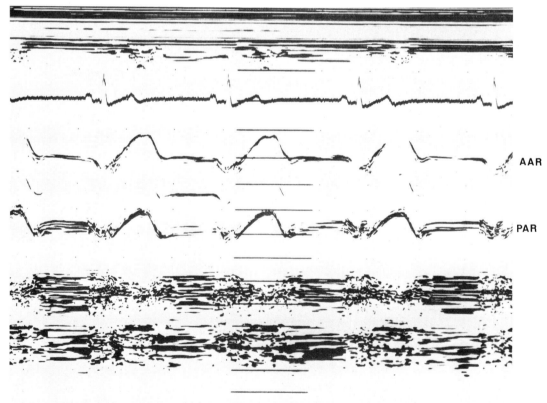

Figure 5–32. Excessive use of gain and reject. Although the walls of the aorta are seen, the aortic valve leaflets have been eliminated (AAR = anterior aortic root; PAR = posterior aortic root).

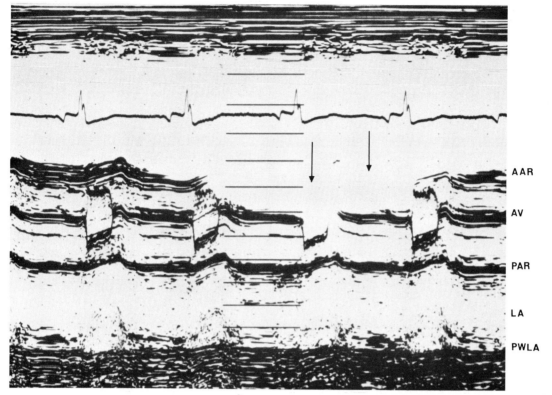

Figure 5–33. Incorrect placement of the TGC curve results in a loss of echoes in the near field (arrows). See Figure 5–3 for correct position of the TGC curve (AAR = anterior aortic root; AV = aortic valve; PAR = posterior aortic root; LA = left atrium; PWLA = posterior wall of left atrium).

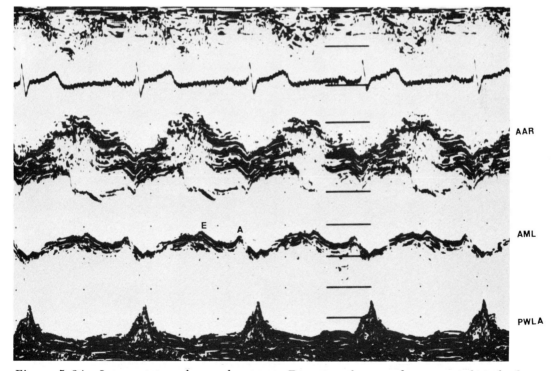

Figure 5–34. Incorrect transducer placement. Directing the transducer too inferiorly from a position too high on the chest results in the following: (1) The motion of the anterior aortic root (AAR) is exaggerated; (2) the characteristic motion of the anterior mitral leaflet (AML), recognized by the E and A waves, is seen in place of the posterior aortic root; and (3) the motion exhibited by the posterior wall of the left atrium (PWLA) is exaggerated as the beam intersects its lowermost portion.

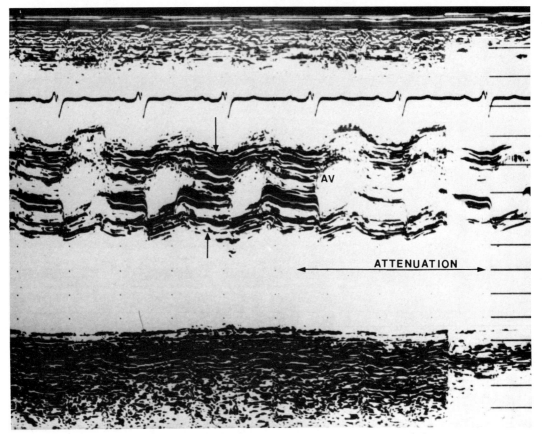

Figure 5–35. Aortic valve infective endocarditis. Multiple parallel echoes are evident during diastole (arrows), but systolic separation of the valve cusps is normal (AV = aortic valve).

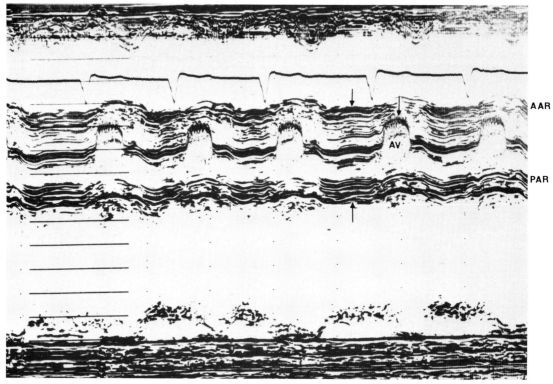

Figure 5–36. Aortic valve vegetations. The box-like configuration of the aortic valve (AV) is apparent, with no restriction to motion of the leaflets. During diastole, there are multiple echoes (arrows), with abnormal thickening of the anterior leaflet during systole (arrow) (AAR = anterior aortic root; PAR = posterior aortic root).

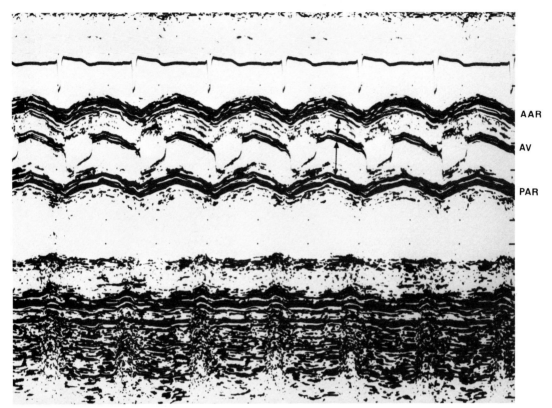

Figure 5–37. Bicuspid aortic valve. The position of the bicuspid leaflets at the time of closure in diastole is off-center (arrows) (AAR = anterior aortic root; AV = aortic valve; PAR = posterior aortic root).

when valve pliability appears normal in spite of very thick leaflet echoes. Gottlieb et al.[21] found that two patients with proven infective endocarditis had dense, highly mobile echo masses within the aortic root in diastole. In four patients in their study, premature mitral valve closure suggested acute aortic regurgitation as well. An example of bacterial endocarditis and vegetations is seen in Figure 5–35. The boxlike configuration of the aortic valve is preserved with no apparent restriction of the leaflets. The outstanding feature is the presence of marked thickening of the valve, as demonstrated by an excessive number of echoes (vegetations) during diastole, with some extra thickening during systole. Figure 5–36 illustrates another patient with bacterial endocarditis and vegetation, evidenced by the thickened echoes during diastole and by marked thickening of echoes on the anterior leaflet during systole.[24]

Bacterial endocarditis may complicate a congenital bicuspid valve, producing aortic regurgitation and large vegetations on the aortic valve or the outflow tract of the left ventricle. Typically, the position of the bicuspid leaflets at the time of valvular closure in diastole is off-center (Fig. 5–37), and multiple echoes caused by valve redundancy as well as calcification and fibrosis are observed during the diastolic phase of the cardiac cycle.

REFERENCES

1. Gramiak R, and Shah PM: Echocardiography of the aortic root. Invest Radiol 3:356–366, 1968.
2. Friedewald VE Jr.: *Textbook of Echocardiography.* Philadelphia, W. B. Saunders Company, 1977.
3. Hernberg J, Weiss B, and Keegan A: The ultrasonic recording of aortic valve motion. Radiology 94:361–368, 1970.
4. Gramiak R, and Shah PM: Echocardiography of the normal and diseased aortic valve. Radiology 96:1, 1970.
5. Feigenbaum H: *Echocardiography.* Philadelphia, Lea and Febiger, 1972.
6. Winsberg F: *Cardiac Ultrasound – The Aortic Valve.* St. Louis, C. V. Mosby Company, 1975.

7. Gramiak R, Shah PM, and Kramer OH: Ultrasound cardiography: Contrast studies in anatomy and function. Radiology 92:939, 1969.

8. Davis RH, Feigenbaum H, Chang S, et al.: Echocardiographic manifestations of discrete subaortic stenosis. Am J Cardiol 33:277–280, 1974.

9. Popp RL, Silverman JF, French JW, et al.: Echocardiographic findings in discrete subvalvular aortic stenosis. Circulation 49:226–231, 1974.

10. Laurenceau JL, Quay JM, and Gagné S: Echocardiography in the diagnosis of subaortic membranous stenosis (Abstr). Circulation (Suppl IV) 48:46, 1973.

11. Davis RH, Feigenbaum H, Chang S, et al.: Echocardiographic manifestation of discrete subaortic stenosis. Am J Cardiol 33:277–280, 1974.

12. Johnson ML, Warren SG, Waugh RA, et al.: Echocardiography of the aortic valve in non-rheumatic left ventricular tract outflow tract lesions. Radiology 112:677–684, 1974.

13. McIntosh HD, Sealy WC, Whalen RE, et al.: Obstruction to outflow tract of left ventricle. Arch Intern Med 110:84–94, 1962.

14. Winsberg F, and Mercer EN: Echocardiography in combined valve disease. Radiology 105:405, 1972.

15. Winsberg F, Gabor GE, Hernberg JG, and Weiss B: Fluttering of the mitral valve in aortic insufficiency. Circulation 41:225, 1970.

16. Edwards JE, and Burchell HB: Endocardial and intimal lesions (jet impact) as possible sites of origin of murmurs. Circulation 18:946–960, 1958.

17. Botvinick EH, Schiller NB, Wickramasekaran R, Klausner SC, and Gertz E: Echocardiographic demonstration of early mitral valve closure in severe aortic insufficiency: Its clinical implications. Circulation 51:836–847, 1975.

18. Friedewald VE, Futral JE, Kinard SA, and Phillips B: Oscillations of the interventricular septum in aortic insufficiency (Abstr). In White D, (Ed.): Ultrasound in Medicine. New York, Plenum Press, 1975, p. 88.

19. Wigle ED, and Labrosse CJ: Sudden, severe aortic insufficiency. Circulation 32:708–720, 1965.

20. Mann T, McLaurin L, Grossman W, and Craige E: Assessing the hemodynamic severity of acute aortic regurgitation due to infective endocarditis. N Engl J Med 293:108–113, 1975.

21. Gottlieb S, Khuddus SA, Bolooki H, et al.: Echocardiographic diagnosis of aortic valve vegetations in candida endocarditis. Circulation 50:826–830, 1974.

22. DeMaria AN, King JF, Salel AF, et al.: Echography and phonography of acute aortic regurgitation in bacterial endocarditis. Ann Intern Med 82:329–335, 1975.

23. Wray TM: Echocardiographic manifestations of flail aortic valve leaflets in bacterial endocarditis. Circulation 52:658–663, 1975.

24. Feigenbaum H: Echocardiography. Philadelphia, Lea and Febiger, 1976.

Chapter 6

THE LEFT ATRIUM

Recording the left atrium is useful in the assessment of mitral valve disease, left atrial tumors, large thrombi originating from a mitral valve prosthesis, and several other forms of acquired and congenital heart disease. Left atrial size can also be a very useful parameter in following any cardiac abnormality in which a change in that measurement may influence the patient's management or prognosis. Fortunately, the anatomical position of the left atrium at approximately the level of the third intercostal space permits easy recording by echocardiography (Fig. 6–1).

A-MODE APPEARANCE

The A-scan appearance of the left atrial chamber is characterized by an echo-free space immediately behind a pair of parallel-moving spikes representative of the aortic root. Approximately 2.0 to 4.0 cm posterior to the posterior wall of the aortic root, the wall of the left atrium appears as a strong signal exhibiting relatively little motion but moving in opposition to the echoes of the aortic root (Fig. 6–2).

M-MODE APPEARANCE

The echo-free area posterior to the aorta represents the chamber of the left atrium. Moving distally and opposite to the motion of the aortic root are the echoes originating from the wall of the left atrium. The motion of the left atrial wall is usually flat, although in its inferior aspect near the mitral orifice, its motion is more anterior in direction during ventricular diastole and posterior during systole. In contrast to the aortic root, which is maximally posterior at the time of mitral closure (during the electrocardiographic QRS complex), the wall of the left atrium is

anterior in position. Near the end of the QRS complex, coinciding with the onset of ventricular systole, the wall begins to move posteriorly. This motion represents the period of atrial filling. The wall reaches its most posterior postion just before mitral valve opening (D point), as the atrium empties during the period of rapid ventricular filling. After this, there is only minimal movement of the left atrial wall in diastole until it moves anteriorly again as the chamber contracts (Fig. 6–3).

RECORDING TECHNIQUE

Just as it is used in locating the aortic root and the aortic valve (see Chapter 5), the mitral valve is also used as a landmark for the detection of the left atrium. When the whip-like motion of the anterior mitral leaflet is recognized on the A-scan, a slight rotation of the transducer superiorly and medially toward the aorta will demonstrate the characteristic parallel-moving double echoes of the aortic root. From this position, a slight rotation of the transducer inferiorly and laterally will bring the aortic valve cusps into view. Great caution should be taken to prevent inferior angulation of the transducer to the point at which the motion of the mitral valve replaces the smooth motion of the aortic root. On such a recording, the anterior wall of the aortic root is obscured, and although the motion pattern of the posterior wall of the aortic root may initially appear normal, closer inspection frequently reveals mitral motion and the presence of a distinct A wave correlating with atrial contraction. This is further evidenced by the appearance of exaggerated contractions of the left atrial wall, which are observed when the ultrasound beam strikes the atrioventricular groove. The presence of

Text continued on page 124

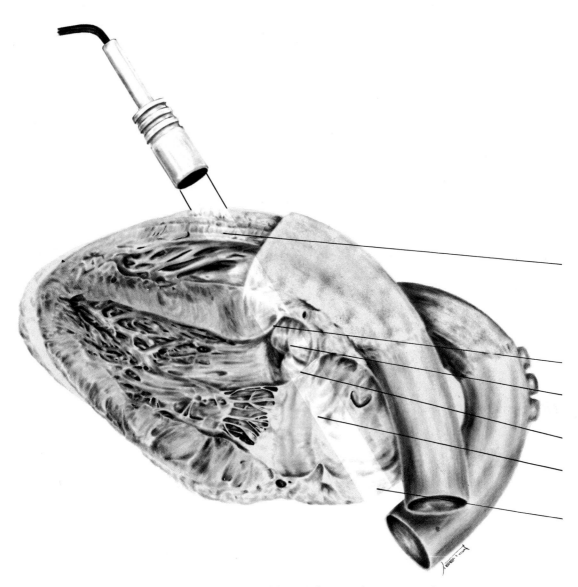

Figure 6–1.   The left atrial chamber is roughly ovoid in configuration. It lies approximately at the level of the third costal cartilage, behind the left half of the sternum, and is oriented superiorly and posteriorly to the other cardiac chambers. Viewed from the left lateral projection, the ultrasound beam is shown passing through the heart and exiting via the left atrium (AWRV = anterior wall of the right ventricle; AAR = anterior aortic root wall; AV = aortic valve; PAR = posterior aortic root wall; LA = left atrium; PWLA = posterior wall of the left atrium).

AWRV

AAR

AV

PAR

LA

PWLA

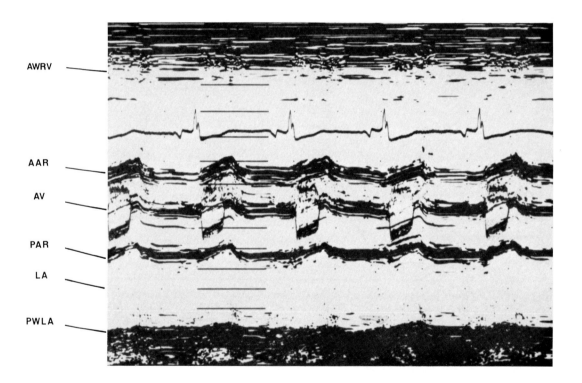

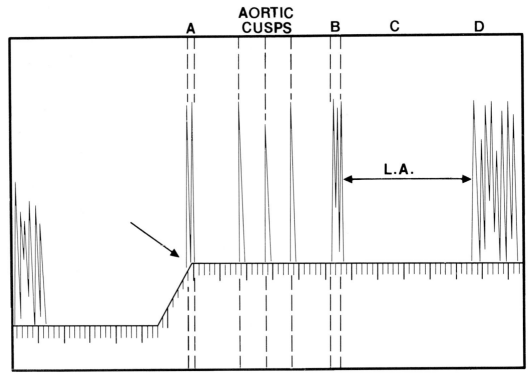

Figure 6-2. A-mode representation of the aortic root and left atrium. The echo designated A represents the anterior aortic root wall; B represents the posterior aortic root wall. The three echoes seen within A and B represent the three aortic valve cusps. The echo-free space designated C represents the left atrial chamber (LA). The close grouping of echoes designated D originates from the left atrial wall. Note the position of the TGC (delay) curve placed against the anterior aortic wall (arrow).

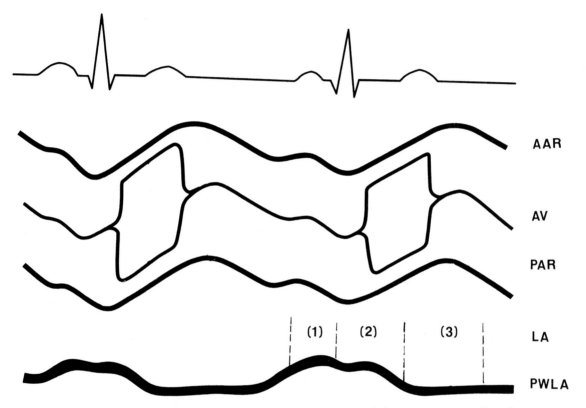

AAR

AV

PAR

(1)   (2)   (3)   **LA**

PWLA

Figure 6–3. In this schematic representation, the motion of the aortic root wall and posterior left atrial wall (PWLA) is purposely exaggerated so that their opposing motion may be better seen. The posterior wall of the left atrium exhibits three phases of motion: (1) anterior movement during atrial systole; (2) posterior movement during ventricular systole; and (3) anterior movement during early ventricular diastole, followed by flattening until the next atrial contraction (AAR = anterior aortic root wall; AV = aortic valve; PAR = posterior aortic root wall; LA = left atrium).

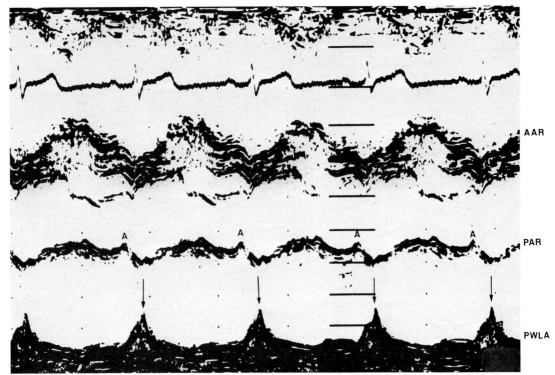

AAR

PAR

PWLA

Figure 6–4.   When the transducer is directed too far inferiorly from the normal aortic valve recording position, the following results will usually occur: (1) the anterior wall of the aortic root (AAR) will
not be clearly demonstrated; (2) the posterior aortic root (PAR) will take on the configuration of mitral
motion, confirmed by the presence of a mitral A wave (A); and (3) the motion of the posterior wall of
the left atrium (PWLA) will be markedly exaggerated (arrows).

exaggerated left atrial wall motion, therefore, is an excellent indicator of incorrect
transducer angulation in recording the left
atrium (Fig. 6–4).

When the aortic root has been identified,
attention should be directed to instrumentation adjustment. The far gain must be adjusted to allow for visualization of the free
movement of the anterior aortic root wall.
The near gain should be adjusted only
enough to allow for the appearance of the
anterior heart wall and right ventricular outflow tract (see Fig. 6–2). The echoes from
the left atrial wall will then appear 2 to 4 cm
posterior to the aortic root. Behind this left
atrial echo is a large group of signals originating from either the lung or the medias-
tinal structures.

LEFT ATRIAL MEASUREMENT

Measurement of the left atrial chamber is
dependent on a positive identification of the
posterior wall of the aortic root and the pos-

terior wall of the left atrium. With the transducer positioned at the fourth intercostal
space and directed superiorly, the left
atrium usually appears behind the mitral
valve. When the mitral valve is recorded
from the third intercostal space, with the
transducer directed farther inferiorly, the
left ventricle is often recorded, making
measurement of the left atrial chamber impossible. For this reason, no measurement
should be attempted when any part of the
normal mitral valve is visualized (Fig. 6–5).

Various ways of measuring the left atrial
dimension are utilized in different laboratories, and each method has its own value
and limitations. Normal values are obviously dependent on the technique elected. The
most commonly used method is that described by Hirata et al.[1] and Brown et al.[2]
The anterior-posterior atrial dimension is
obtained by measuring the distance from
the anterior edge of the posterior aortic root
wall to the strong endocardial echo of the
posterior left atrial wall at the end of ventricular systole (end of the electrocardiogra-

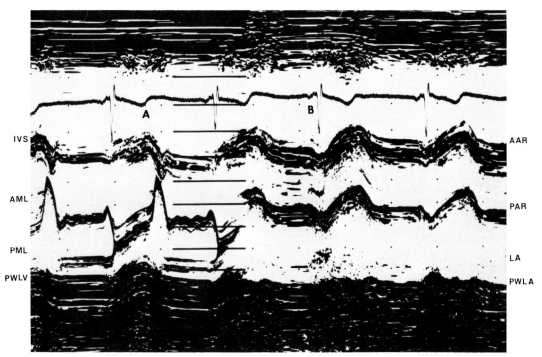

Figure 6–5.   As the ultrasonic beam makes the transition from the region of the mitral valve (MV) and left ventricular posterior wall (PWLV) up to the region of the aorta, the following echocardiographic changes occur. Area A is characterized by the echoes from the interventricular septum (IVS), the anterior leaflet of the mitral valve (AML), the posterior leaflet of the mitral valve (PML), and the left ventricular posterior wall (PWLV). On the sweep toward the aorta (B), the interventricular septum is replaced by echoes from the anterior aortic root wall (AAR). The mitral valve loses its characteristic "M" shape and is replaced by echoes from the posterior aortic root wall (PAR). The echo-free space of the left atrial chamber (LA) is visible immediately proximal to the posterior aortic wall. Note the differences in patterns of motion between the left ventricular posterior wall and the less mobile posterior left atrial wall (PWLA).

phic T wave). It is during this phase of the cardiac cycle that the left atrium exhibits its maximum size (Fig. 6–6). It is also acceptable to measure from the posterior edge of the posterior aortic root wall to the left atrial wall. In the majority of cases, however, the anterior edge of the posterior aortic root wall provides a more clearly defined echo from which to measure. Accuracy is further insured when some portion of the aortic valve cusps is visualized between the margins of the aortic root. It is from the aortic valve recording position that the ultrasound beam passes through the right ventricular outflow tract, the aortic root and valve cusps, the left atrial cavity, and the left atrial wall (Fig. 6–1).

It should be mentioned that the presence of inert, intracavitary echoes ("ghost echoes") arising from within the left atrium should not be mistaken for the posterior left atrial wall when measurements are made. The origin of these echoes is in dispute, but they are frequently seen in the presence of a thickened mitral annulus. They have, however, also been attributed to the pulmonary veins (Fig. 6–7).

Determining Absolute Left Atrial Size

In the presence of any one of several cardiac abnormalities, the size of the left atrium is a factor in assessing both the severity and the progression of the disease. Prior to the introduction of ultrasound diagnosis, radiological methods were generally employed for assessing the size of this chamber. As well as being potentially hazardous to the patient, however, this method often produced misleading results.[3]

A major advantage of the echocardiogram over routine chest x-rays is that a true internal left atrial dimension can be obtained. Although this measurement represents only one dimension of the ovoid-elliptical chamber, the left atrium tends to enlarge in

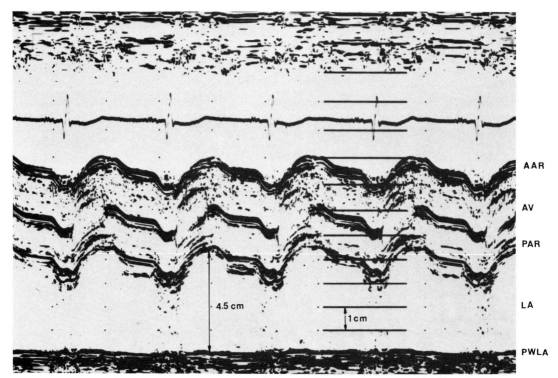

Figure 6–6. The left atrial dimension (LA) is obtained by measuring the distance from the posterior aortic root wall (PAR) to the posterior left atrial wall (PWLA). This measurement is obtained at the end of ventricular systole, immediately following the T wave of the electrocardiogram. Utilizing the calibrated vertical 1-cm lines, the left atrial dimension is approximately 4.5 cm (AAR = anterior aortic root; AV = aortic valve).

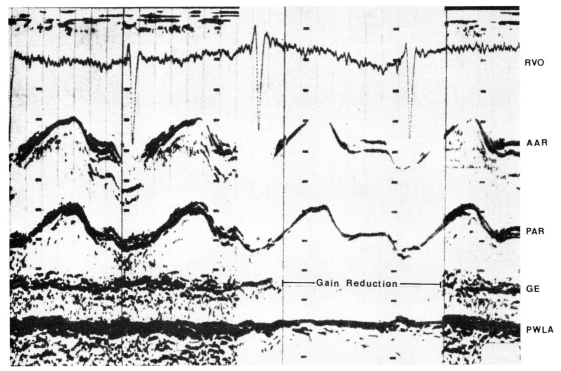

Figure 6–7.   The presence of intracavity echoes or a "ghost echo" (GE) within the left atrium may be mistaken for the posterior left atrial wall (PWLA). This echo disappears with an increase in the attenuation. In measuring the left atrial chamber, the ghost echo should be ignored (RVO = right ventricular outflow tract; AAR = anterior aortic root wall; PAR = posterior aortic root wall).

all directions, and one dimension will reflect any change in size.

To date, although the left atrial dimension can be measured with a great degree of accuracy from the echocardiogram, a form of compensation is necessary in establishing standardized size. For example, in a patient with a small heart, enlargement of the small left atrium may go undetected because the left atrial size measures within the normal range of 2.1 cm to 4.0 cm; likewise, left atrial dimensions falling outside the normal range may be found in the patient with a large absolute cardiac size. Thus, what may be a normal left atrial size for one patient may also be abnormal for another. It has been recognized that left atrial size will be equivalent, roughly, to aortic root size, but it is necessary to compensate accurately for variations in normal cardiac size. In their original work, Hirata and his associates correlated the size of the left atrium with the body surface area.[1] The correlation of angiographic data and the mean left atrial dimension measured from the echocardiograms of normal subjects was shown to be 3.1 cm ±

0.5 cm, with a range of 1.8 to 4.0 cm. When divided by body surface area, the normal range was 1.2 to 2.0 cm per M^2 (Fig. 6–8). This method remains the basis for differentiating between the normal and the enlarged left atrium.

Another method of comparing absolute left atrial dimensions with parameters that reflect normal cardiac size is described by Brown et al.[2] Their method is based upon the assumption that regardless of absolute cardiac size, the anatomical dimensions of the normal heart are proportional and that this relationship is constant from subject to subject (see Figure 6–9). Because the fibrous portion of the aortic root can be recorded accurately with echocardiography and does not enlarge as the result of common forms of cardiac disease, Brown and his associates compared the echocardiographic size of the aortic root at end-diastole with the end-systolic dimension of the left atrium in 170 patients.[2] In 50 subjects, their results demonstrated a consistent left atrial–aortic root (LA–AO) ratio in the range of 0.87 to 1.11 in patients without hemodynamic

Nomogram for Calculating the Body Surface Area of Adults

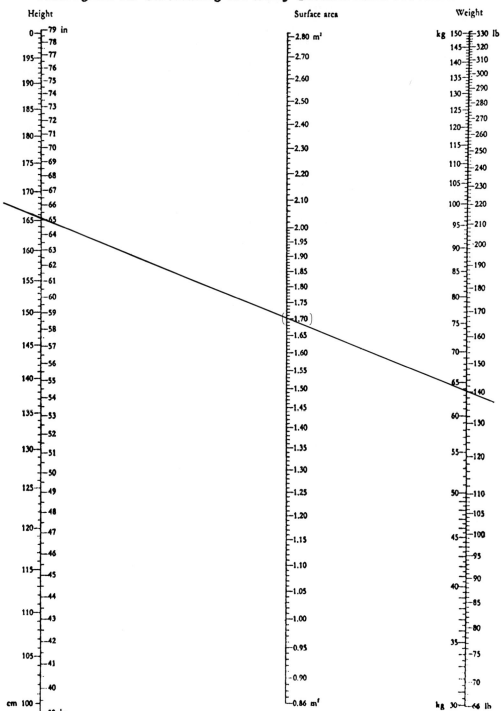

Figure 6–8. (A) To utilize the BSA (Body Surface Area) chart, it is necessary to know the patient's height and weight. The surface area is then obtained by placing a ruler from the patient's height in the left column to the patient's weight (line). The surface area is the number intersected in the center column. Note a surface area of 1.70 M² in a patient with a height of 5'5 (65″) and a weight of 140 lbs. The formula for this calculation is: $cm/M^2 = \dfrac{LA\ diameter}{surface\ area}$. On the echocardiographic recording (B), the left atrial dimension (LAD) at end-systole, measured from the posterior aortic root wall (PAR) to the posterior left atrial wall (PWLA), is approximately 4.1 cm. Dividing this number by the surface area (1.70 M²), this recording illustrates a slight atrial enlargement of 2.4 cm/M².

Illustration continued on opposite page

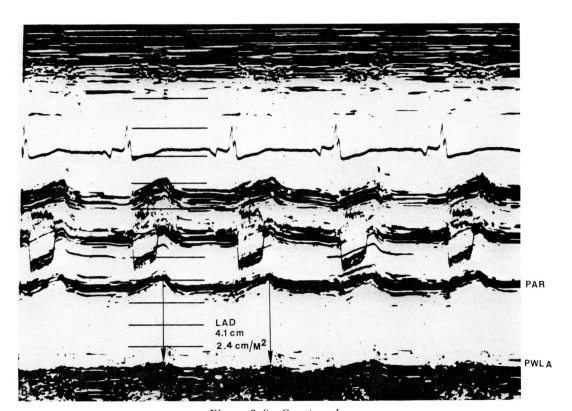

PAR

LAD
4.1 cm
2.4 cm/M^2

PWL A

Figure 6–8   Continued.

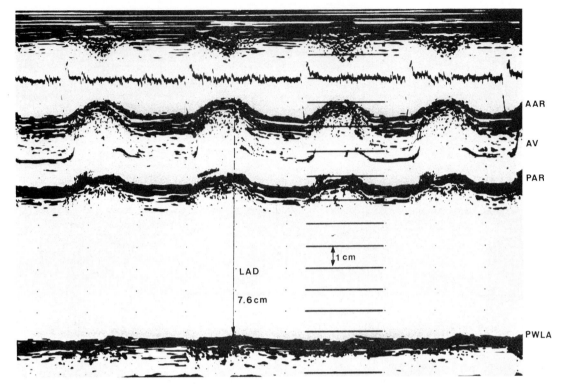

Figure 6–9. Left atrial enlargement usually occurs as a result of mitral valve disease or left ventricular failure. The magnitude of left atrial enlargement is one index of the severity of disease. In this echocardiographic recording, the left atrial dimension (LAD) is approximately 7.6 cm, whereas the aortic root measures approximately 3.2 cm (dotted line). This recording was obtained from a relatively small person, and when adjusted for body surface area (BSA chart — Figure 6–8) (1.72 cm/M²), the absolute left atrial size is 4.4 cm/M², considerably above the normal upper limit of 2.0 cm/M² (AAR = anterior aortic root wall; AV = aortic valve; PAR = posterior aortic root wall; PWLA = posterior left atrial wall).

cause for left atrial enlargement. The mean dimension of the left atrium was 3.2 cm, with a range of 2.3 to 4.4 cm. In 80 patients, LA–AO ratios of 1.17 or greater were found to be indicative of left atrial enlargement. In 40 patients with isolated aortic valve disease, dilatation of both the aortic root and the left atrium resulted in LA–AO ratios of less than 1.17 in some patients.

In cases of severe mitral valve calcification, frequently seen in mitral stenosis, the left atrial dimension will be distinctly enlarged (Fig. 6–10).

Instrumentation

The accurate assessment of left atrial size by the echocardiogram is mainly dependent upon recording technique. Excessive use of the expand and/or depth control, for example, will cause distortion of the echoes emanating from the posterior left atrial wall (Fig. 6–11). Furthermore, improper transducer angulation may give a false impression of exaggerated left atrial wall motion and size (Fig. 6–12). When such a recording is produced, it is necessary to return to the original recording position and to re-record the movement from the aortic root to the posterior left atrial wall, with only slight posterior angulation of the transducer head.

Overuse of the gain control will increase attenuation, and echoes from the posterior left atrial wall will be obscured. When this occurs, the recording will be unsatisfactory for estimation of the left atrial measurement (Fig. 6–13). Because of the importance of this dimension in the echocardiographic diagnosis, it is advisable to make several recordings of the left atrial chamber and

Text continued on page 138

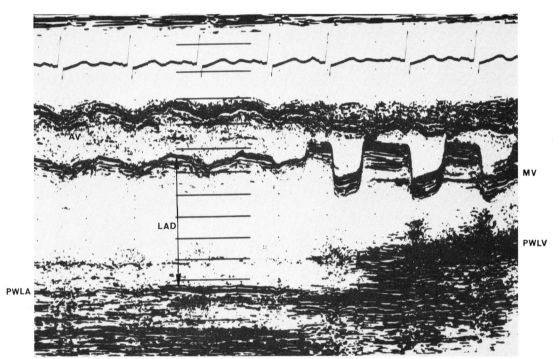

Figure 6–10.   Left atrial dilation in mitral stenosis. On this sector scan from the aortic root to the highly stenotic mitral valve (MV), the left atrial wall (PWLA) is displaced posteriorly relative to the position of the posterior left ventricular wall (PWLV). The left atrial dimension measures 6 cm. The aortic valve (AV) appears to be pliable, although not clearly seen.

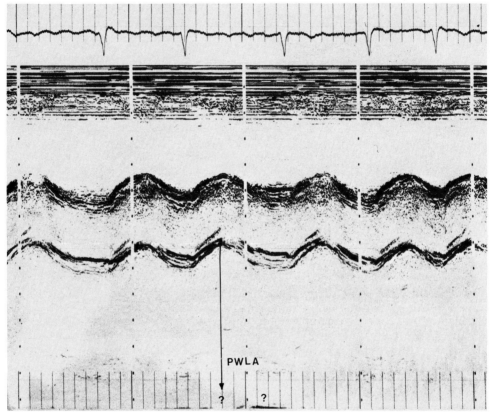

Figure 6–11.   With excessive use of the depth and/or expand control, the recording is extended too far, limiting the view of the posterior left atrial wall (PWLA). Although some echoes are visible in the vicinity of the posterior left atrial wall, their origin is uncertain, and the left atrial chamber cannot be reliably measured.

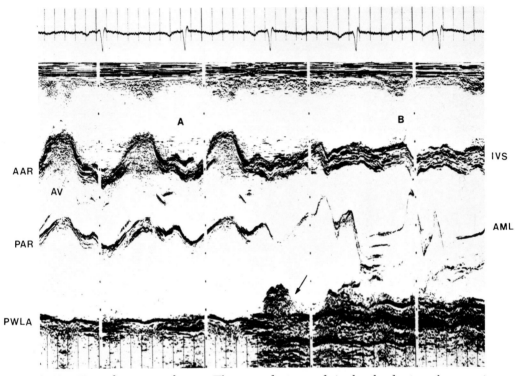

Figure 6-12. Transducer angulation. The area designated A clearly depicts the anterior aortic root (AAR), portions of the aortic valve cusps (AV), the posterior aortic root (PAR), and the characteristic subtle motion of the posterior left atrial wall (PWLA). In area B, the transducer has been aimed more posteriorly from the original recording position. This results in replacement of the anterior aortic wall echo by those characteristic of the interventricular septum (IVS). No portion of the aortic valve is visible. The echo originating from the posterior aortic root is replaced by echoes of the anterior mitral valve leaflet (AML). This is confirmed by the presence of distinct mitral motion. Note the exaggerated concentrations of the left atrial wall in area B (arrow) versus the less mobile motion of the left atrial wall in area A.

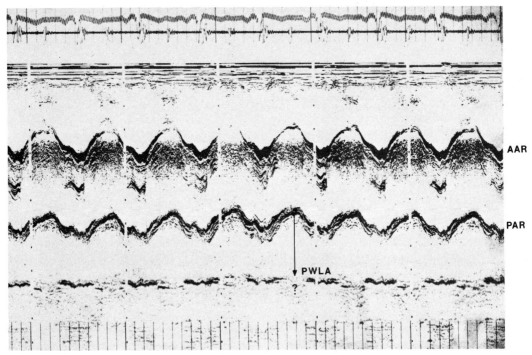

Figure 6–13. Because of the increased attenuation, the echoes of the posterior left atrial wall (PWLA) are not clearly shown, and therefore the left atrial chamber cannot be measured accurately (arrow) (AAR = anterior aortic root; AV = aortic valve; PAR = posterior aortic root).

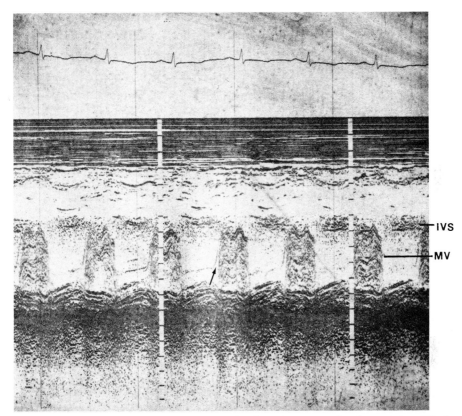

IVS

MV

Figure 6–14.   Left atrial myxoma. The anterior leaflet of the mitral valve (MV) is filled with many interfaces of multiple echoes representative of the tumor as it passes through the valve orifice. The decreased E-F slope of the mitral valve is due mainly to the myxoma's obstruction of the inflow of blood into the left ventricle. Note the echo-free space (arrow) that is seen momentarily after the opening of the mitral valve prior to entry of the mass into the mitral orifice (IVS = interventricular septum).

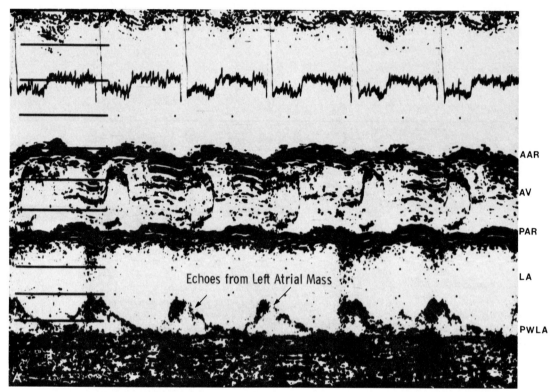

Figure 6–15. (A) Extensive mitral valve calcification is not unusual in severe long-lasting mitral disease and may be seen adjacent to the wall of the left atrium. Note the abnormal protrusions arising along the posterior wall of the left atrium (PWLA) (arrows). Identification of calcium formation necessitates precise use of instrumentation. It must also be pointed out that such calcification can be mistaken for the previously discussed "ghost echoes."

Illustration continued on opposite page

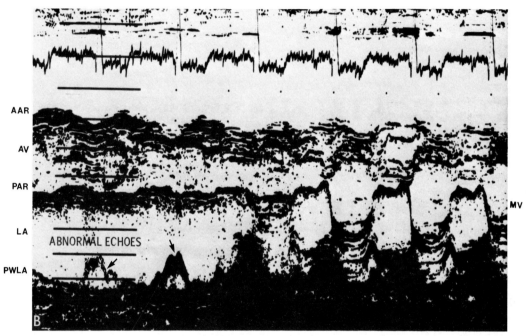

Figure 6–15 Continued.   (B) On the sector scan from the aortic root to the mitral valve (MV), the abnormal protrusions, representative of calcific material, continue from the posterior wall of the left atrium (PWLA) (arrows), where it is reflected within the mitral valve. The echo-filled mitral valve bears a close resemblance to an atrial myxoma. Note the strong, heavy echoes posterior to the mitral valve (AAR = anterior aortic root; AV = aortic valve; PAR = posterior aortic root).

walls to ensure that an accurate echocardio-gram is available for calculation of the absolute left atrial dimension.

Left atrial size can be assessed in the patient with a grossly enlarged left atrium using the suprasternal notch approach (see Chapter 2). The aorta, the right pulmonary artery, and the left atrium can be identified by directing the transducer inferiorly and toward the heart from the suprasternal notch position. In normal cases, the average dimension of the left atrium is 4.1 cm using this technique.

Left Atrial Mass

The echocardiographic detection of a left atrial myxoma is principally contingent upon the tumor's extending through the mitral orifice during diastole (mitral valve opening) (Fig. 6–14). The motion of the mitral valve is altered principally in that the E-F slope is reduced as a result of decreased flow across the obstructed mitral orifice and because the tumor physically prevents normal partial closure of the valve in mid-diastole.[4] Furthermore, the posterior mitral leaflet may be difficult or impossible to record in some patients as it becomes obscured by the dense tumor echoes.[5] Although rare, the formation within the left atrium of a calcified thrombus that protrudes through the mitral orifice can produce very similar characteristics (Fig. 6–15). It should be mentioned that the detection of a thrombus formation within the left atrium by ultrasound is unreliable.[6] This is due mainly to the fact that the acoustic impedance of a thrombus is similar to that of unclotted blood, unless the thrombus is highly organized and calcified.

REFERENCES

1. Hirata T, Wolfe SB, Popp RL, Helmen CH, and Feigenbaum H: Estimation of left atrial size using ultrasound. Am Heart J 78:43–52, 1969.
2. Brown RO, Harrison DC, and Popp RL: An improved method for echographic detection of left atrial enlargement. Circulation 50:58–64, 1974.
3. Hawley RR, Dodge HT, and Graham TP: Left atrial volume and its changes in heart disease. Circulation 34:989, 1967.
4. Bodenheimer MM, Moscovitz HL, Pantazopoulous J, and Donoso E: Echocardiographic features of experimental left atrial tumor. Am Heart J 88:615–620, 1974.
5. Friedewald VE Jr.: Textbook of Echocardiography. Philadelphia, W. B. Saunders Company, 1977, p. 133.
6. Tallury VK, and DePasquale NP: Ultrasound cardiography in the diagnosis of left atrial thrombus. Chest 59:501–503, 1971.

Chapter 7

THE LEFT VENTRICLE

Recording the left ventricle is perhaps the most difficult part of the routine echocardiographic examination, primarily because high-quality posterior wall echoes and septal echoes must be recorded simultaneously. Routine recording of the left ventricle permits evaluation of the following:

1. Detection of abnormal wall motion.
2. Determination of left ventricular wall thickness.
3. Measurement of the internal dimensions of the left ventricle in systole and diastole. These dimensions are used for the calculation of left ventricular volume, stroke volume, cardiac output, ejection fraction, and circumferential muscle fiber shortening velocity.

ANATOMY

The left ventricle is the largest of the cardiac chambers. It is surrounded by thick, muscular walls measuring 8 to 16 mm, approximately two to three times the thickness of the right ventricular walls. The left ventricle is roughly oval in shape and forms the apex of the heart. The left ventricle is inferior to the left of the atrium. Its function is to receive oxygenated blood from the left atrium and to eject it through the aorta to the peripheral tissues. Thus, the left ventricle must generate relatively high pressures in order to overcome the resistance of the peripheral vessels.

The anterior and medial wall of the left ventricle is the interventricular septum. Most of the ventricular septum is muscular and has approximately the same thickness as the left ventricular free wall. Both the septum and posterior basal free wall are simultaneously recorded on the standard echocardiographic recording of the left ventricle.

The chamber of the left ventricle contains the leaflets of the mitral valve and the chordae tendineae, which extend from the papillary muscles. The anteromedial leaflet of the mitral valve is suspended in such a manner that when it is open, in diastole, it separates the left ventricular cavity into an inflow tract and an outflow tract.[1] The inflow tract is formed by the mitral annulus and both valve leaflets and their chordae tendineae. The outflow tract is surrounded by the inferior surface of the anteromedial mitral leaflet, the interventricular septum, and the left ventricular wall (Fig. 7–1).

THE POSTERIOR WALL

A-Mode Appearance

On the A-mode, the posterior wall of the left ventricle is represented on the oscilloscope as the most posterior moving cluster of spikes, ranging from 3 to 5 cm posterior to the interventricular septum. Characteristically, these echoes are all of similar amplitude. They move in unison, anteriorly during systole and posteriorly during diastole, and have a total width of about 0.6 cm to 1.2 cm (Fig. 7–2).

M-Mode Appearance

When seen on the M-mode, the posterior left ventricular wall in the normal subject

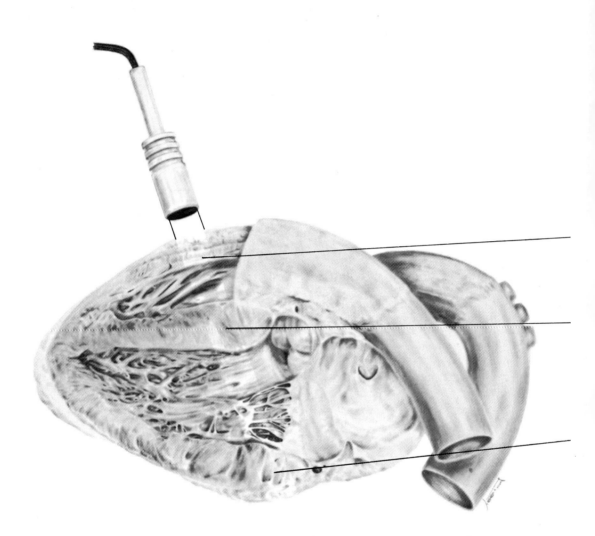

Figure 7–1. The left ventricle. The ultrasonic beam intersects the muscular interventricular septum and the posterior left ventricular wall below the posterior mitral leaflet (AWRV = anterior wall of right ventricle; IVS = interventricular septum; PWLV = posterior wall of left ventricle).

Illustration continued on opposite page

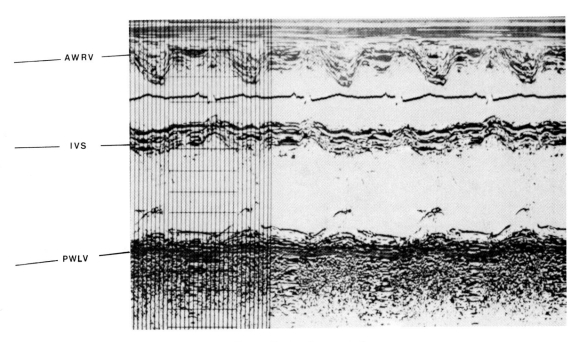

Figure 7–1. *Continued.*

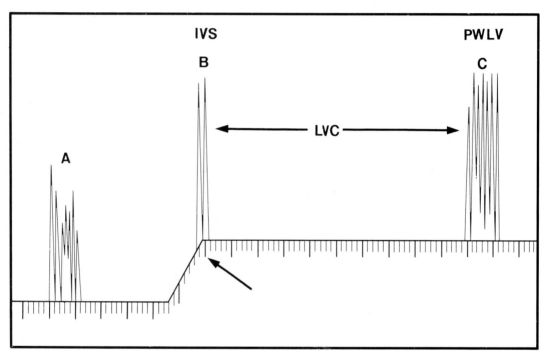

Figure 7-2. In this A-mode schematic representation, the left ventricular chamber (LVC) (arrow) is identified as follows: The echoes designated A are representative of the anterior heart wall. B represents the echoes originating from the interventricular septum (IVS). (Note the placement of the TGC curve (arrow), allowing full visualization of both the anterior and posterior wall of the septum.) The cluster of echoes designated C arise from the posterior left ventricular wall (PWLV).

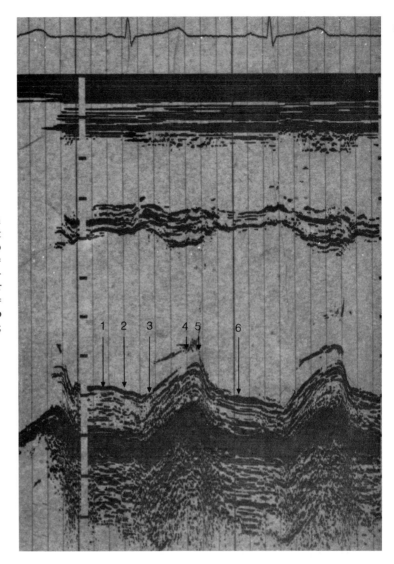

Figure 7–3. Motion pattern of the normal posterior left ventricular wall (PWLV). (1) to (2) = atrial filling; (2) to (3) = period of isovolumic contraction; (3) to (4) = ventricular ejection phase; (4) to (5) = isovolumic relaxation; (5) to (6) = period of early diastole; (6) to (1) = mid-diastole.

appears as a heavy band of synchronously moving echoes. The motion pattern is easily recognizable because contraction of the posterior wall appears as a series of rounded projections during ventricular systole (Fig. 7–3).

There are three distinct echo components of the posterior wall of the left ventricle. From the inside out, they are the following:

1. The endocardial surface appears as a relatively faint echo that moves anteriorly during ventricular systole. Of particular importance is that it exhibits a more rapid rate of anterior motion than the other structures in this region. During diastole, it has a rapid posterior excursion followed by a slower movement posteriorly.

2. The myocardium, located between the endocardium and epicardium, appears as echoes of lesser intensity than the other left ventricular wall echoes.

3. The echoes of the epicardial-pericardial interface are strong and are reflected as echoes denser than those of the myocardium (anterior) and the lung (posterior). The edge of the epicardial-pericardial interface is most obvious when a pericardial effusion is present. This echo also moves anteriorly during ventricular systole, but at a slower rate than the endocardial echo (Fig. 7–4).

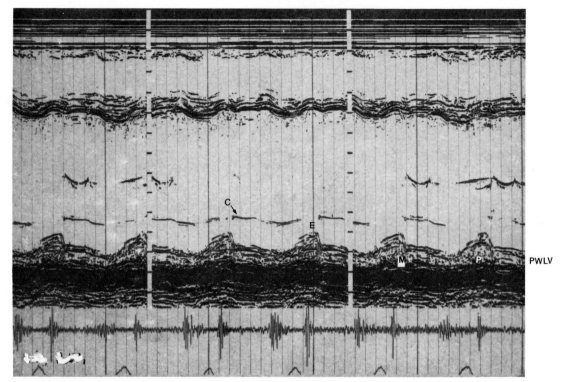

Figure 7–4. The posterior wall of the left ventricle (PWLV). A chordal echo (C) is seen as a slowly moving echo anterior to the endocardium. The endocardial echo (E) is fainter and shows the greater systolic motion. The myocardium (M) immediately behind the endocardium contains low-intensity echoes, while the epicardial-pericardial interface (P) produces the most intense echo.

RECORDING TECHNIQUE

After the patient is positioned comfortably, preferably on his left side, a good starting point for transducer placement is in the mitral valve position, in the fourth intercostal space, close to the sternum. It is wise to use the mitral valve as a landmark when recording the posterior wall of the left ventricle, because the posterior wall should be recorded just below the posterior mitral leaflet and above the posteromedial papillary muscle.

Following visualization of the mitral valve, rotation of the transducer laterally and slightly inferiorly will result in diminished mitral motion. Minute angulation further inferiorly should continue until the systolic excursion of the posterior wall of the left ventricle becomes more pronounced and the mitral valve disappears from view. There are no set or standardized control settings for recording the posterior wall of the left ventricle, but it should be emphasized that sensitivity control (gain and reject) adjustments are critical and should be kept at a minimal level for identification of pericardial-epicardial echoes. When these echoes appear, the gain can be decreased until the echoes originating from the endocardium come into view (Fig. 7–5).

Because minute errors in angulation and misidentification of posterior wall echoes can easily result in mismeasurement of the left ventricular internal dimension, some words of caution must be interjected at this point. It is possible to mistake the posterior chordae tendineae for the endocardium, because their echoes exhibit a similar motion pattern just anterior to the endocardial echo. The echoes originating from the chordae tendineae will be of stronger intensity than the endocardial echoes and will exhibit less motion during systole. These echoes appear suspended anterior to the echoes of the posterior wall of the left ventricle (Fig. 7–6). Also, when closely evaluated, the echoes originating from the chordae tendineae can

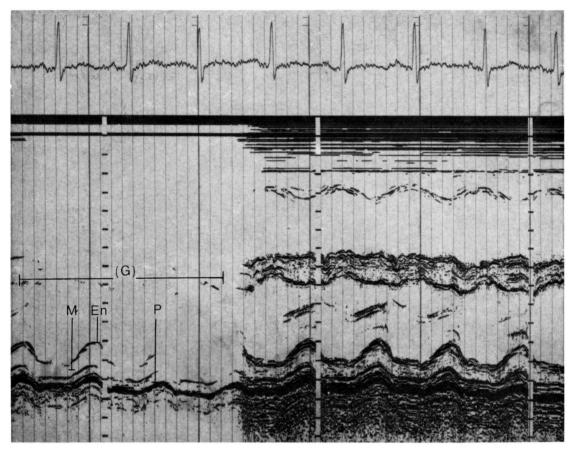

Figure 7–5. Gain study. With reduced gain (G), the three tissue components that compose the posterior wall are distinctly visualized. From top to bottom, they are the endocardium (En), the myocardium (M), and the pericardium (P).

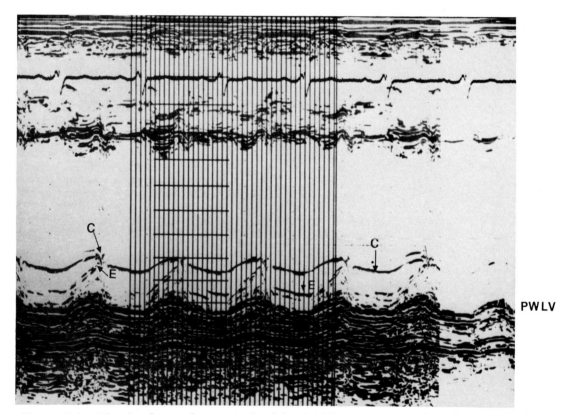

Figure 7–6.   The chordae tendineae. A chordal echo (C) is seen as a relatively heavy band with only slight anterior systolic excursion. The endocardial echo (E) is less intense and exhibits the greatest systolic motion (PWLV = posterior wall of the left ventricle).

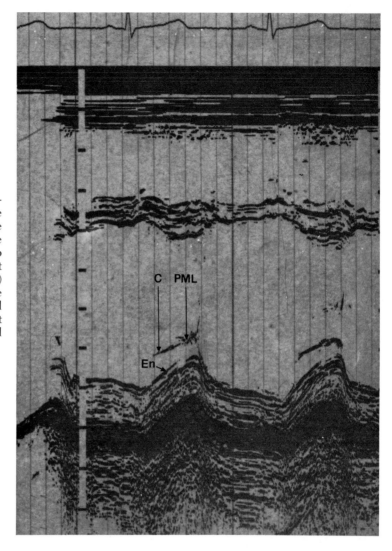

Figure 7–7. In this echocardiographic recording, the echoes originating from the chordae tendineae (arrow) are seen attached to the faint echo of the posterior mitral leaflet (arrow). The endocardium (En) is seen directly posterior to the chordal echo (C = chordal echo; PML = site of attachment of chorda to posterior mitral leaflet).

be seen attached to the leaflets of the mitral valve (Fig. 7–7).

If the transducer is directed too far inferiorly, the result is usually a reduction of the left ventricular dimension as the transducer beam is directed more toward the apex. Other changes in angulation can cause a loss of a clear endocardial echo, making accurate measurement of the left ventricular dimension difficult and resulting in the appearance of reduced contractility. This could be mistaken for poor left ventricular function (Fig. 7–8). Before recording, a visual check should clearly demonstrate (1) endocardial and epicardial surfaces of the posterior left ventricular wall and (2) the anterior and posterior edges of the interventricular septum. The reject and gain controls should be set to eliminate all low-intensity echoes, but care must be taken to preserve the low-intensity endocardial echo.

The aortic root also serves as an excellent landmark in identifying the left ventricular walls. When the aortic root has been identified on the A-mode, the TGC should be adjusted to rest against the leading edge of the anterior wall of the aortic root. After slight angulation of the transducer laterally and inferiorly, the wave form of the echo from the anterior aortic root will be observed to merge into the interventricular

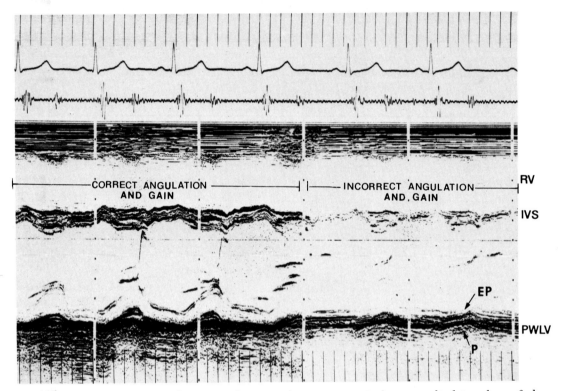

Figure 7–8. Incorrect transducer angulation and excessive gain have resulted in a loss of clear endocardial echoes. This is evidenced in this M-mode representation in which only the epicardial (Ep) and pericardial echoes are visualized. Because the left ventricular chamber is measured from the endocardium to the posterior wall of the interventricular septum (IVS), this error in transducer angulation prevents an accurate assessment of left ventricular dimension (RV = right ventricle; PWLV = posterior wall of the left ventricle).

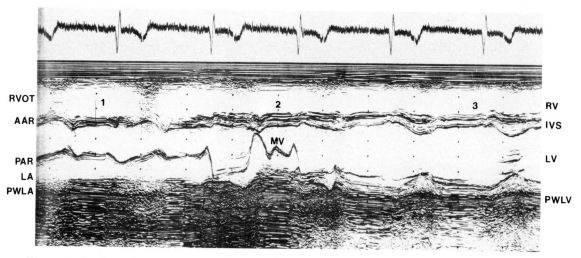

Figure 7–9. Scan from the aorta to the mitral valve (MV) and left ventricle (LV). Using the aortic root as a landmark and sweeping downward to the left ventricle involves first establishing the plane of axis of the structures to be recorded. This is performed by scanning from the aortic root (1) downward to optimal motion of the mitral valve (2). Once this plane has been established (roughly a line from the right shoulder to the left iliac crest), the transducer is then directed inferiorly from a point just below the tip of the mitral leaflets until the motion of the posterior left ventricular wall (PWLV) is identified (3) (RVOT = right ventricular outflow tract; AAR = anterior aortic root; PAR = posterior aortic root; LA = left atrium; PWLA = posterior wall of the left atrium; IVS = interventricular septum).

septum. As the transducer is directed more inferiorly, the echo from the posterior aortic root will gradually diminish. Accordingly, mitral motion will then be observed. Further angulation of the transducer laterally and inferiorly will reveal an absence of the mitral valve as the left ventricular chamber and the endocardial surface of the posterior left ventricular wall comes into view (Fig. 7–9).

Although it takes considerable practice to learn to perform the sector scan (sweep), this technique provides a standardized approach to the echocardiographic recording. In recording the left septal and posterior walls of the left ventricle, it is important to recognize that only one structure at a time can be identified and that a standard sequence must be followed. For example, when using the aortic root as a landmark, the interventricular septum should be identified first, then the left ventricular wall. At that point, control settings (TGC) should be ad-

justed, first to enhance septal echoes, then to record the posterior ventricular wall echoes. Mastery of this technique will provide distinct recordings of all structures.

LEFT VENTRICULAR WALL THICKNESS

The importance of determining the thickness of the posterior wall of the left ventricle is twofold: (1) it provides a valuable parameter in the assessment of left ventricular muscle mass; and (2) this measurement plays a significant role in the echocardiographic diagnosis of various forms of cardiac hypertrophy.

Wall thickness is measured on the echocardiogram from the endocardial echo to the epicardial-pericardial echo during late diastole or at the R wave of the electrocardiogram.[2, 4] During this diastolic phase, the

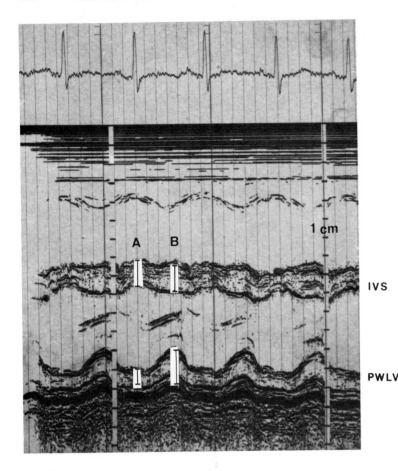

Figure 7-10. At the R wave of the electrocardiogram, both the width of the interventricular septum (IVS) and the posterior left ventricular wall (PWLV) measure approximately 1.2 cm (A). Following the T wave of the electrocardiogram, the posterior wall reaches its most anterior displacement. At this point in the cardiac cycle, both the interventricular septum and the posterior wall are maximally thickened, each measuring approximately 1.8 cm (B) in this example. The vertical calibration markers are 1 cm apart.

normal posterior wall thickness ranges from 0.8 cm to 1.3 cm. During ventricular systole, both the posterior wall and the interventricular septum thicken to approximately equal width (Fig. 7–10).[5, 6] The normal width of the posterior left ventricular wall in systole ranges from approximately 1.3 cm to 1.9 cm.

LEFT VENTRICULAR DIMENSIONS

As with the other segments of the echocardiographic tracings, it is an excellent practice for the person doing the echocardiographic examination to calculate the left ventricular measurements. Awareness of what is necessary for accurate calculations will lead to the production of high-quality recordings. Otherwise, what may appear technically accurate will prove to be inadequate for valid measurement from the recording.

At end-systole (ESD), just prior to the T wave of the electrocardiogram, the posterior wall reaches its peak anterior excursion, and ventricular chamber size is measured from the endocardial echo to the left ventricular edge of the septum. During this phase, the septum is usually near its most posterior point of contraction. (Maximum posterior displacement of the septum usually slightly precedes the maximum posterior wall anterior position.)

The left ventricular size at end-diastole (EDD) is measured at the time of the onset of the QRS complex of the electrocardiogram, from the posterior edge of the septum to the endocardial echo of the posterior wall (Fig. 7–11). The end-diastolic measurement is the single most reliable echocardiographic measurement of left ventricular size. Depending on such factors as flow rate and diastolic filling time, the end-systolic and end-diastolic dimensions will vary. In the event that there is a major variance, it is always a good idea to measure several recordings, making positive identification of

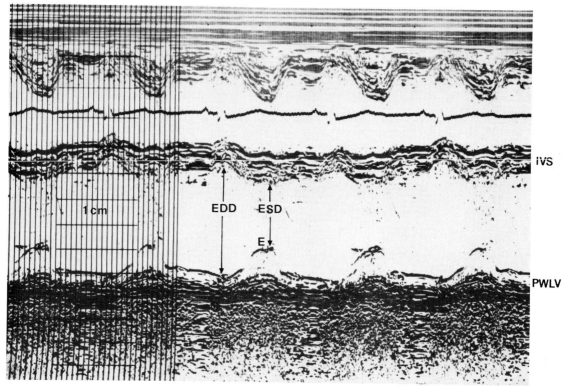

Figure 7–11. The end-diastolic dimension (EDD) is measured at the time of the electrocardiographic R wave, from the left ventricular edge of the septum to the endocardial (E) echo of the posterior wall. The end-systolic dimension (ESD) is measured at the time of maximal anterior excursion of the posterior wall (following the T wave of the electrocardiogram), from its endocardial echo to the left ventricular edge of the interventricular septum (IVS) (PWLV = posterior wall of the left ventricle).

the interventricular septum and endocardial echoes. It should be interjected at this point that both the end-systolic and end-diastolic measurements should be obtained from the same set of cardiac cycles for accurate determination of left ventricular function.

VENTRICULAR VOLUMES

The ability to calculate left ventricular volumes from the chamber dimensions during the cardiac cycle follows characterization of the normal and abnormal clinical states.[7, 8] Such determinations make possible the measurement of left ventricular stroke volume,[9] estimation of ejection fraction and cardiac output, and evaluation of velocity of circumferential fiber shortening.

In the normal left ventricle, cubing the systolic dimension (Sd^3) approximates the blood volume of the left ventricle at the

end of systole. Cubing the diastolic dimension (Dd^3) approximates the blood volume at the end of diastole. The volumes determined in this way have shown a significant correlation with angiographic volume estimations.[10, 11] It should be emphasized that the use of the cube function of the echocardiographic minor axis is an accurate predictor of volumes only in ventricular chambers of normal or near-normal size.[12] Some other factors that invalidate these methods for volume estimation include:

1. Localized areas of akinesia or dyskinesia of any portion of the ventricle, including the septum, as symmetrical contraction is lost.[11]

2. Abnormal septal motion, as in left bundle branch block and right ventricular volume overload (Fig. 7–12). In the event of chamber enlargement, the volume size will be progressively overestimated as the left ventricular dimensions increase. The error

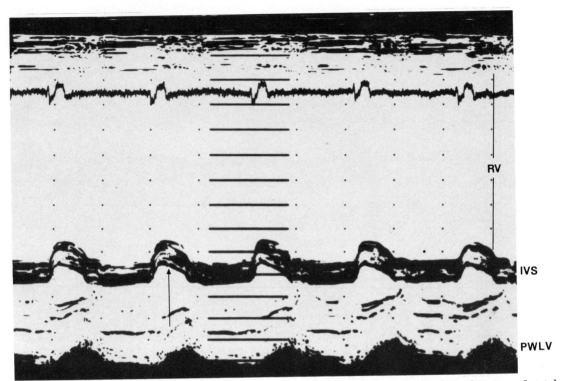

Figure 7–12.   Paradoxical septal motion in right ventricular volume overload. In this case of atrial septal defect, the interventricular septum (IVS) moves anteriorly (arrow) during ventricular systole, paralleling the motion of the posterior left ventricular wall (PWLV). The right ventricle (RV) is grossly dilated. In this recording, left ventricular volume estimation by echocardiography cannot be accurately determined.

occurs because the long axis of the chamber becomes less than twice the minor axis determination as the ventricle assumes a shape that is more nearly spherical instead of cylindrical.[11, 14]

Stroke Volume

Stroke volume (SV) is the amount of blood ejected from the ventricle in one cardiac cycle. This measurement is determined by calculating the difference between the end-systolic volume (ESV) and end-diastolic volume (EDV). This is expressed as

$$SV = EDV - ESV$$

Popp and Harrison found that there was an excellent correlation between the echo stroke volume and that derived by the Fick method.[15] As a precaution, it should be emphasized that here, too, in the presence of a severely enlarged left ventricle, using this calculation in the estimation of stroke volume will result in an overestimated volume.

Ejection Fraction

The ejection fraction (EF) is the percentage of blood present in the ventricle at the end of diastole that is ejected during ventricular systole. As stroke volume (SV) was determined by subtracting ESV from EDV, ejection fraction is determined by dividing the stroke volume by the end-diastolic volume.[10] This is expressed as

$$EF = \frac{SV}{EDV}$$

The ejection fraction is an index of the efficiency of the left ventricle in handling the volume of blood delivered to it. The ejection fraction decreases as the myocardium fails.[16]

Cardiac Output

The amount of blood pumped by the heart in one minute, termed the cardiac output (CO), is a product of stroke volume (SV) and heart rate (HR). This is represented by the equation

$$CO = HR \times SV$$

Thus, as the body's oxygen requirement rises, as during exercise, the cardiac output will increase by means of the increasing heart rate and stroke volume.

Velocity of Circumferential Fiber Shortening

In addition to ejection fraction and cardiac output, the mean velocity of circumferential fiber shortening (V_{CF}, expressed in circumferences per second) provides yet another parameter of ventricular function. V_{CF} is directly related to cardiac muscle function and thus may furnish information about ventricular performance (myocardial contractility) that cannot be obtained from a consideration of ejection fraction alone.[17] Investigators have shown that determination by cineangiography of the mean velocity of shortening of the minor internal circumference equator of the left ventricle correlates with normal or reduced myocardial contractility.[18, 20, 23] The V_{CF} is computed by assuming that the left ventricular diameter measured is equal to the true diameter of the left ventricular minor axis. The formula for deriving the mean V_{CF}, which is normally greater than 1.10 circumference per second, is as follows:

$$\text{Mean } V_{CF} = (EDD - ESD)/(EDD \times ET)$$

where EDD = End-diastolic dimension
ESD = End-systolic dimension
ET = Ejection time of the left ventricle.[19]

The ET can be determined by measuring the time from the QRS peak of the electrocardiogram to the maximum anterior displacement of the posterior wall in systole, minus 50 sec, to correct for the pre-ejection period.[23] Calculation of the ET may also be determined by measuring the time from the beginning of posterior wall movement anteriorly to its maximal anterior position.[16]

A number of diseases that affect myocardial contractility have been found to alter the V_{CF}.[23] From the formulae, it is apparent that a shortened left ventricular ejection time and a reduced ejection fraction both result in an abnormal decrease in the V_{CF}. Examples of this are mitral stenosis and left ventricular failure.[17] Conversely, when the ejection time is shortened but the ejection fraction is increased in such diseases as IHSS without failure, the V_{CF} may be increased.

Left Ventricular Wall Velocity — Systole

The mean and peak velocities of posterior wall motion have been used as measures of left ventricular contractility.[17] In the normal ventricle, the velocity of the endocardial surface is greater than that of the epicardium. In left ventricular dysfunction, they may be almost equal. The posterior wall velocity in systole is the rate (cm/sec) at which the endocardial surface moves anteriorly during ventricular systole. This measurement is taken from the beginning of contraction to the peak systolic anterior position (Fig. 7–13). In one study, the normal maximal systolic endocardial velocity was 6.2 ± 1.4 cm/sec with a mean systolic endocardial velocity of 4.1 ± 0.7 cm/sec.[21] Following exercise, in this same study, a significant increase was seen in the mean posterior wall velocity.

Other investigators have found there to be a poor correlation between posterior wall velocity and other parameters of left ventricular function during systole. Some of these include ejection fraction, the mean velocity of circumferential fiber shortening (V_{CF}), and the ratio of pre-ejection period to left ventricular ejection time (PEP/LVET).[22, 23]

In the presence of cardiac arrhythmias, variations in posterior wall velocity are most apparent. Fluctuations in the left ventricular volume in these cases are probably the cause for the posterior wall changes from beat to beat.[23]

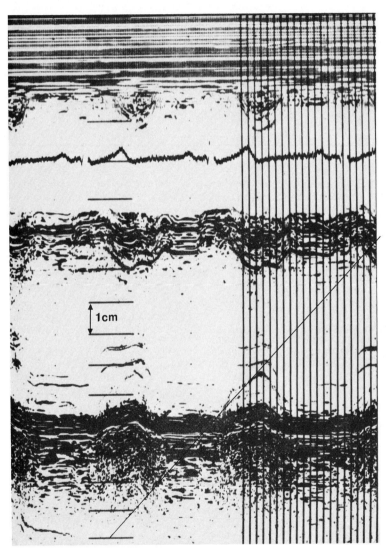

Figure 7–13. Left ventricular wall velocity. The velocity of the posterior wall measurement is determined from the beginning of contraction to the peak systolic anterior position (tangent line). In this echocardiographic illustration, the systolic endocardial velocity measures approximately 6.1 cm/sec.

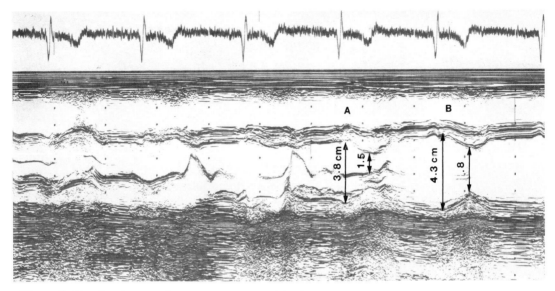

Figure 7–14. In plane A, the measurements of the left ventricular cavity have been made too high in the ventricle at the level of the mitral valve. The measurements were made from an echo most probably originating from the mitral apparatus or cordae tendineae rather than from the endocardium. This results in a smaller measurement than in plane B, which is the correct plane from which to make the left ventricular measurement.

Left Ventricular Wall Velocity — Diastole

Fogelman et al. proposed that following systolic contraction, the rate of posterior excursion of the left ventricular posterior wall is a function of myocardial relaxation.[21] They found that the maximal diastolic endocardial velocity was 18 ± 3 cm/sec and that the mean early diastolic endocardial velocity was 9.4 ± 1.7 cm/sec. During exercise, these values were found to increase, but in the presence of ischemia they were abnormally reduced.

Although the left ventricular velocity both in systole and in diastole may be helpful in characterizing generalized diseases such as cardiomyopathies, it is necessary that further studies in this area be performed before definite conclusions can be made.

COMMON ERRORS THAT PRODUCE VARIATIONS IN LEFT VENTRICULAR DIMENSION

A successful echocardiographic recording of the left ventricle is more dependent on the expertise of the technologist than on any other single factor. Although the echoes from the posterior left ventricular wall can be easily recorded in most patients, the endocardial surface of the posterior wall may not be recorded if the proper instrumentation and transducer angulation are not used. This is especially true when recording echoes from the interventricular septum. In addition to technical expertise, the ultrasonic equipment must have sensitive gain controls, so that the septum can be "tuned in" individually without affecting echoes from the more distal structures. Figures 7–14 to 7–17 illustrate some of the various errors that may be produced when recording the left ventricular chamber.

MYOCARDIAL DISEASE AND THE MITRAL VALVE

As the flow into the left ventricle becomes restricted owing to such diseases as hypertrophic cardiomyopathy and coronary artery disease, the flow rate across the mitral valve is also reduced. This results in the E and A points exhibiting a similar amplitude of excursion (Fig. 7–18). In some instances, it is not uncommon for the mitral E point to actually show less excursion than the A point.

In congestive cardiomyopathy, because of the massive dilation of all the chambers, both mitral leaflets are extremely easy to record. Normally, the mitral valve is posi-

Text continued on page 165

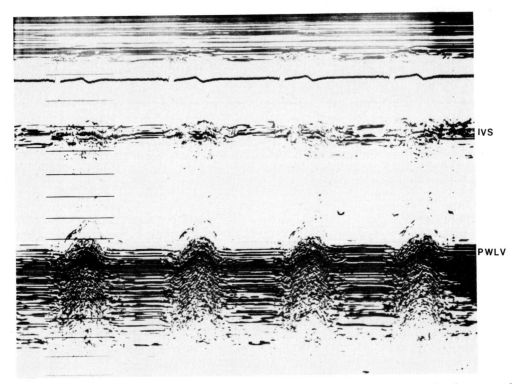

Figure 7–15.   Incorrect transducer angulation. The ultrasound beam is not completely perpendicular to the structures being recorded. This results in indistinct interfaces such as the right and left sides of the interventricular septum and the endocardial and epicardial echoes of the left ventricular posterior wall. Accurate measurement of the left ventricular chamber is difficult although some general idea as to its relative size can be ascertained (IVS = interventricular septum; PWLV = posterior wall of the left ventricle).

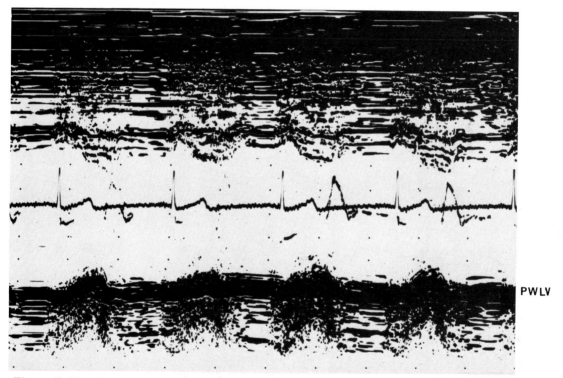

Figure 7–16. Instrumentation errors that obscure the septal echoes and cause non-visualization of the endocardium. Owing to excessive use of the near gain, the right side or anterior portion of the septum cannot be clearly delineated. Furthermore, because of an increased reduction in the far gain, the endocardial surface of the posterior left ventricular wall (PWLV) is absent.

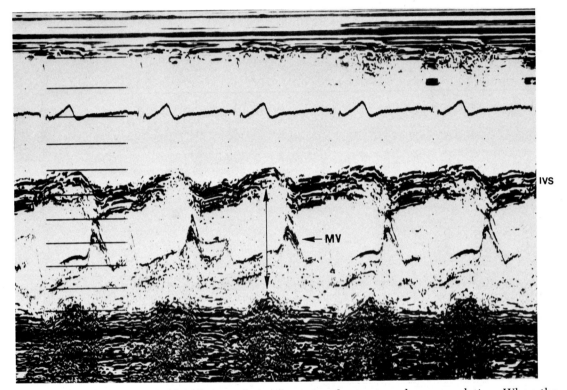

IVS

← MV

Figure 7–17. (A) Erroneous paradoxical septal motion due to transducer angulation. When the echo beam intersects the interventricular septum (IVS) so high that the mitral valve (MV) is seen in its entirety, an erroneous diagnosis of "paradoxical" septal motion may be made (arrow).

Illustration continued on opposite page

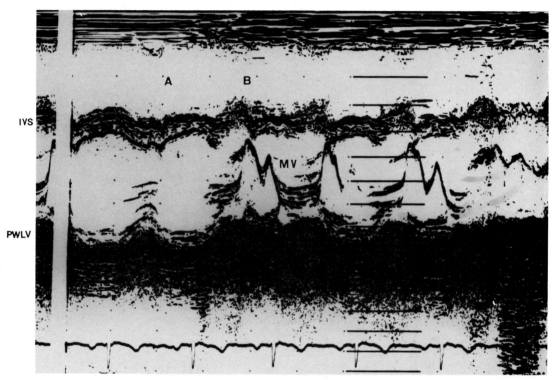

Figure 7–17 Continued.   (B) Scan from the left ventricle to the mitral valve (MV). Within the body of the left ventricular chamber, the interventricular septum (IVS) moves posteriorly toward the posterior wall of the left ventricle (PWLV) during systole *(A)*. Conversely, when the mitral valve is recorded, the septum moves anteriorly *(B)*.

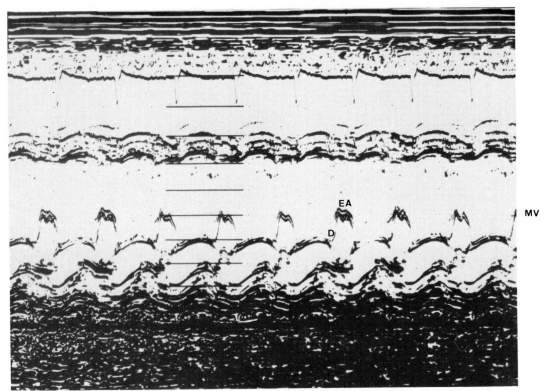

Figure 7-18. The overall small appearance of the mitral valve (MV) is caused by reduced flow into the left ventricle and accordingly across the mitral valve. In addition to the reduced amplitude of the D-E excursion, note the similarity in amplitude of the E and A waves.

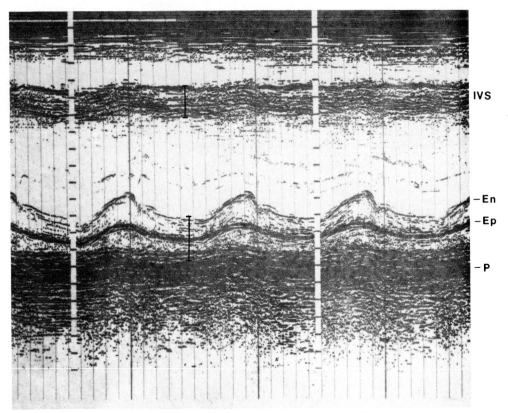

Figure 7-19. An abnormally thickened posterior left ventricular wall measuring 2.5 cm. This thickness could be due to coagulated matter occupying the pericardial space or left ventricular hypertrophy. The septum is also thickened at 1.8 cm. Paradoxical septal motion is demonstrated (IVS = interventricular septum; En = endocardium; EP = epicardium; P = pericardium).

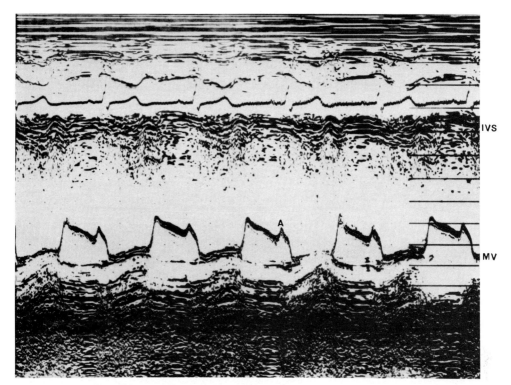

Figure 7–20. Reduced left ventricular compliance. The E-F slope of the mitral valve (MV) is reduced to approximately 20 mm/sec, the result of decreased rate of blood flow into the left ventricle. The valve, however, appears pliable, as manifested by the distinct A wave. Furthermore, the valve leaflets show no evidence of being thickened (IVS = interventricular septum).

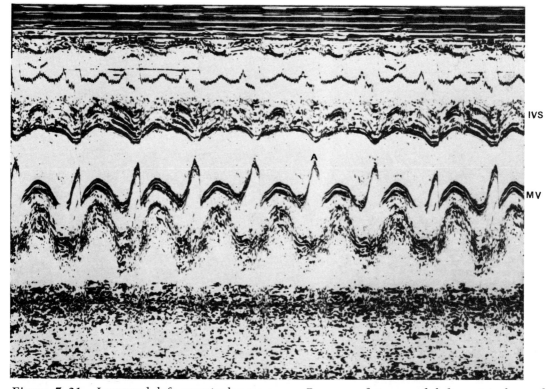

Figure 7–21. Increased left ventricular pressure. Because of increased left ventricular end-systolic pressure, the mitral valve (MV) E wave is absent. Mitral valve opening occurs only after atrial contraction (*A*). Note the large pericardial effusion present (IVS = interventricular septum).

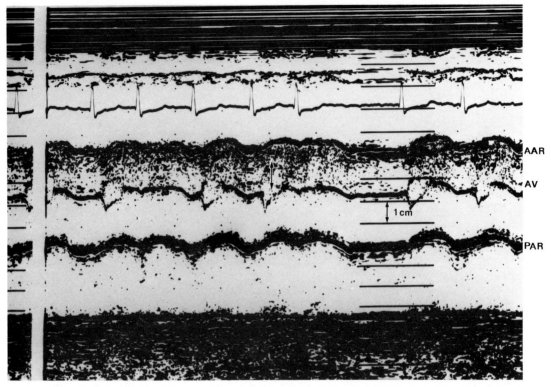

Figure 7–22. The effect of low cardiac output on the aortic valve. The abbreviated opening of the aortic valve (AV) is due to poor left ventricular function and decreased stroke volume. The valve measures approximately 1.3 cm (AAR = anterior aortic root; PAR = posterior aortic root).

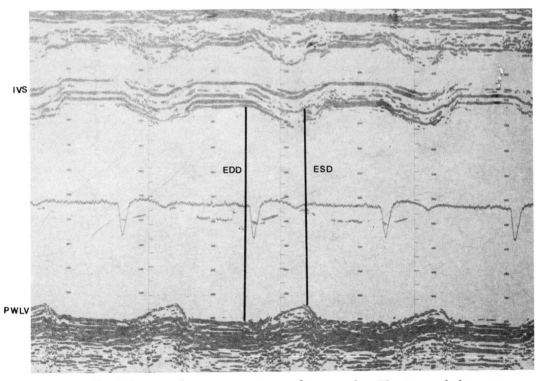

Figure 7–23. The left ventricle in congestive cardiomyopathy. The internal dimensions are markedly increased (ESD = 7.5 cm, EDD = 8.9 cm). The posterior left ventricular wall (PWLV) exhibits diminished amplitude of excursion, as does the interventricular septum (IVS).

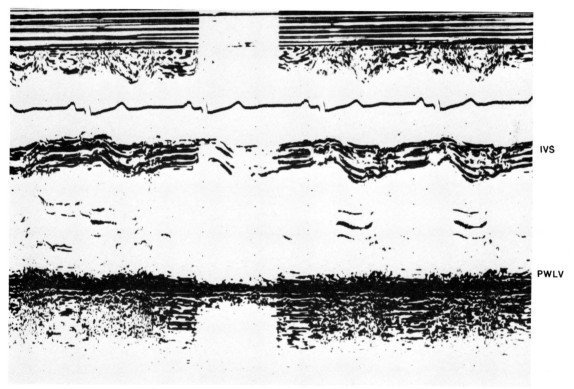

IVS

PWLV

Figure 7–24.   Posterior left ventricular wall myocardial infarction. There is little or no discernible posterior wall (PWLV) motion during ventricular systole. The septum (IVS) exhibits a normal motion. A 12-lead electrocardiogram substantiated the posterior wall infarction.

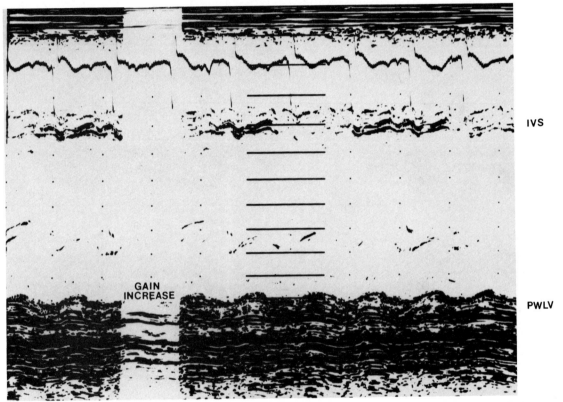

Figure 7–25. Ventricular aneurysm with thrombus formation. The left ventricular internal dimension is markedly increased, with diminished posterior wall (PWLV) excursion and paradoxical septal (IVS) motion. Post mortem, the apparent disproportionate thickness of the posterior wall (gain decrease) was found to be part of a large calcified thrombus.

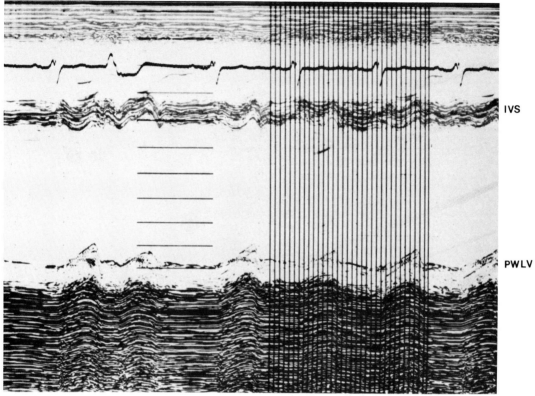

Figure 7-26. Ventricular aneurysm. The left ventricular internal dimension is markedly increased. The posterior ventricular wall (PWLV) shows moderately good contractility, while the septum (IVS) demonstrates very little motion (hypokinetic).

tioned in close apposition to the posterior wall echo. As the ventricle distends in left ventricular failure, the mitral echoes become removed from the posterior wall. Also, the reduced flow across the valve causes the small opening of both the E and A waves to take on a "fishmouth" appearance (Fig. 7-19). Various examples demonstrating the effects of myocardial disease on mitral motion and other cardiac structures are seen in Figures 7-20 to 7-26.

REFERENCES

1. Walmsley R, and Watson H: The outflow tract of the left ventricle. Br Heart J 28:435, 1966.
2. Feigenbaum H, Popp RL, Chip JN, and Kaine CL: Left ventricular wall thickness measured by ultrasound. Arch Intern Med 121:391, 1968.
3. Popp RL, Schroeder JS, Stinson EB, Shumway NE, and Harrison DC: Ultrasonic studies for the early detection of acute cardiac rejection. Transplantation 11:543, 1971.
4. Troy BL, Pombo JF, and Rackley CE: Ultrasonic measurements of left ventricular wall thickness and mass. Circulation 43:480, 1971.
5. McDonald IG, Feigenbaum H, and Chang S: Analysis of left ventricular wall motion by reflected ultrasound: Application to assessment of myocardial function. Circulation 46:14–25, 1972.
6. Bennett DH, Evans DW, and Ray VJ: Echocardiographic left ventricular dimensions in pressure and volume overload: Their use in assessing aortic stenosis. Br Heart J 37:971–977, 1975.
7. Dodge HT, and Baxley WA: Hemodynamic aspects of heart failure. Am J Cardiol 22:24, 1968.
8. Dodge HT, and Baxley WA: Left ventricular volume and mass and their significance in heart disease. Am J Cardiol 23:528, 1969.
9. Dodge HT, Hay RD, and Sandler H: Angiographic method for directly determining left ventricular stroke volume in man. Circ Res 11:739, 1962.
10. Pombo JF, Troy BL, and Russel RO Jr.: Left ventricular volumes and ejection fraction by echocardiography. Circulation 43:480, 1971.
11. Gibson DG: Estimation of left ventricular size by echocardiography. Br Heart J 35:128–134, 1973.
12. Murray JA, Johnston W, and Reid JM: Echocardiographic determination of left ventricular dimensions, volumes and performance. Am J Cardiol 30:252–257, 1972.
13. Redwood DR, Henry WL, and Epstein SE: Evaluation of the ability of echocardiography to measure acute alterations in left ventricular volume. Circulation 50:901–904, 1974.
14. Fortuin NJ, Hood WP Jr., Sherman ME, and Craige E: Determination of left ventricular volumes by ultrasound. Circulation 44:575–584, 1971.
15. Popp RL, and Harrison DC: An atraumatic method for stroke volume determination using ultrasound (Abstr). Clin Res 17:258, 1969.
16. Fortuin NJ, Hood WP, and Craige E: Evaluation of

left ventricular function by echocardiography. Circulation 46:26–35, 1972.

17. Fortuin NJ, Hood WP Jr., Sherman ME, and Craige E: Determination of left ventricular volumes by ultrasound. Circulation 44:575, 1971.

18. Belenkie I, Nutter DO, Clark DW, McGraw DB, and Raizner AE: Assessment of left ventricular dimensions and function by echocardiography. Am J Cardiol 31:755–762, 1972.

19. Cooper RH, O'Rourke RA, Karliner JS, Peterson KL, and Leopold GR: Comparison of ultrasound and cineangiographic fiber shortening in man. Circulation 46:914–923, 1972.

20. Quinones MA, Gaasch WH, and Alexander JK: Echocardiographic assessment of left ventricular function with special reference to normalized velocities. Circulation 50:42–51, 1974.

21. Fogelman AM, Abbasi AS, Pearce ML, and Kattus AA: Echocardiographic study of the abnormal motion of the posterior left ventricular wall during angina pectoris. Circulation 46:905–913, 1972.

22. Ludbrook P, Karliner JS, London A, Peterson KL, Leopold GR, and O'Rourke RA: Posterior wall velocity: An unreliable index of total left ventricular performance in patients with coronary artery disease. Am J Cardiol 33:475–482, 1974.

23. Friedewald VE Jr.: *Textbook of Echocardiography.* Philadelphia, W.B. Saunders Company, 1977.

Chapter 8

THE INTERVENTRICULAR SEPTUM

Because of its anatomical position, the interventricular septum is an essential landmark in the measurement of the individual cardiac chambers and is of great importance in echocardiographic "sweeping" from one structure to another. In addition, septal motion and septal thickness are valuable parameters in the detection of cardiac abnormalities. It is therefore essential that the interventricular septum be accurately identified and recorded.

ANATOMICAL FEATURES

The heart is a four-chambered muscular organ that is divided from top to bottom by a septum. The upper cardiac chambers, the atria, are divided right from left by the interatrial septum. The right and left lower chambers, the ventricles, are separated by the interventricular septum. The interventricular septum, an essentially muscular structure, is an outgrowth of the ventricular wall itself and forms a common border of the two ventricles. It is roughly triangular in shape, with the base of the triangle at the level of the aortic cusp at approximately the third intercostal space. It is composed entirely of muscle, except at the top, where a small membranous segment helps to support the right and noncoronary aortic cusps. The muscular portion of the septum has approximately the same thickness as the posterior wall of the left ventricle and does not lie in any single plane, but it appears to exhibit a slight longitudinal twisting motion.

The interventricular septum, including most of its membranous segment, forms the right and anterior border of the left ventricle. The posterior cusp of the tricuspid valve attaches itself to the membranous septum. The continuity of the septum with these valves can be appreciated when executing the echocardiographic technique of "sweeping" from one structure to another.

ECHOCARDIOGRAPHIC FEATURES

A-Mode

While the techniques of identifying and recording the various cardiac structures seem to vary with individual ultrasound facilities, we have found that, as with all the cardiac structures, the best technique for recording the interventricular septum is to use primarily the A-mode. A simultaneous M-mode display is then used for fine control adjustments prior to recording.

The A-mode appearance of the interventricular septum can be recognized as two close together but distinct spikes of equal amplitude. These two signals are located in a relatively anterior position, or to the left of the oscilloscope, and represent the right and left edges of the interventricular septum (Fig. 8–1). When compared to the wide range of motion exhibited by the mitral valve, the A-mode appearance of septal motion is remarkably subtle.

The interventricular septum is most readily identified in two projections: (1) the plane of the anterior leaflet of the mitral valve and (2) in the left ventricle. When the transducer is directed toward the body of

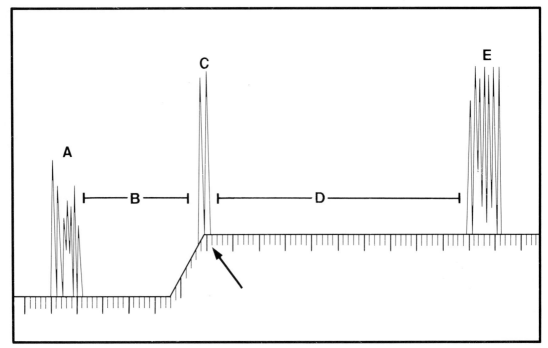

Figure 8–1. A-mode representation of the interventricular septum. The cluster of echoes designated A originates from the anterior wall of the right ventricle. The echo-free space designated B is the right ventricular chamber. The echoes designated C represent the interventricular septum. The echo-free space designated D is the left ventricular chamber. The close grouping of echoes designated E originates from the posterior wall of the left ventricle. Note the position of the TGC (delay) curve positioned against the anterior portion of the interventricular septum (arrow).

the left ventricle, the ultrasound beam intersects the portion of the septum that separates the right and left ventricles called the muscular septum. The muscular septum is seen as a double band of echoes that moves for the most part posteriorly during ventricular systole and anteriorly during diastole. The anterior portion of the muscular septum represents the right ventricular side, while the posterior portion represents the left ventricular side. The left ventricular aspect of the septal wall moves more posteriorly than its right ventricular side. Thus, in addition to its posterior movement, the muscular septum also thickens during ventricular systole (Fig. 8–2).[1]

When the transducer is directed more superiorly toward the anterior leaflet of the mitral valve, the ultrasound beam can intersect the upper portion of the interventricular septum within or adjacent to the membranous septum. The membranous septum forms part of the anteromedial border of the left ventricular outflow tract and is continuous with the anterior wall of the aortic root. For this reason, its normal motion is similar to that of the aortic root walls, i.e., anterior in systole and posterior in diastole. This motion is opposite that of the muscular septum, and this becomes apparent in a continuous echocardiographic scan of the septum from the membranous to the muscular portion (Fig. 8–3). The systolic anterior septal motion sometimes seen in the mitral valve projection should not be mistaken for an abnormally moving septum, hence the importance of executing a complete sweep from the aortic valve to a point inferior to the mitral valve leaflets. An additional characteristic pattern of the membranous septum in the mitral valve projection is a concise, posterior "notching" that occurs immediately after the E point of the mitral valve (Fig. 8–4). Frequently, in cases of mitral stenosis, the septal notch is grossly exaggerated (Fig. 8–5).

RECORDING TECHNIQUE

The echocardiographic determination of left ventricular volumes and the derived

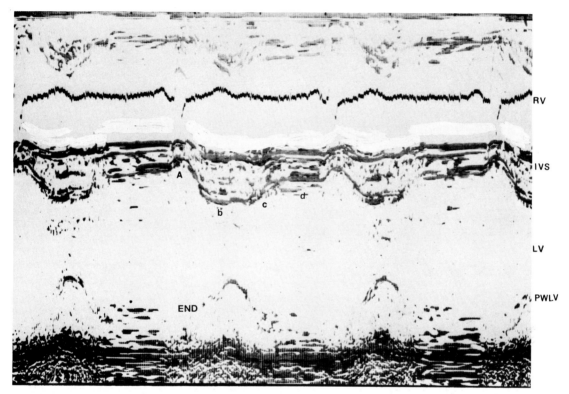

Figure 8–2. The muscular septum (IVS). Following the electrocardiogram inscription of the P wave in diastole, the septum moves abruptly anteriorly. This motion continues until just after the onset of the QRS complex in systole (a). It then exhibits a rather rapid motion posteriorly that continues during most of the systole, opposing the motion of the posterior wall of the left ventricle (PWLV). During this part of the cardiac cycle (systole), the septum thickens into the left ventricle (b). Following systole (end of the T wave), the septum moves anteriorly to its diastolic position (c). This anterior motion is attributed to septal relaxation. During late diastole, the septum is relatively motionless (d). This is the point where septal thickness should be measured (RV = right ventricle; LV = left ventricle; END = endocardium).

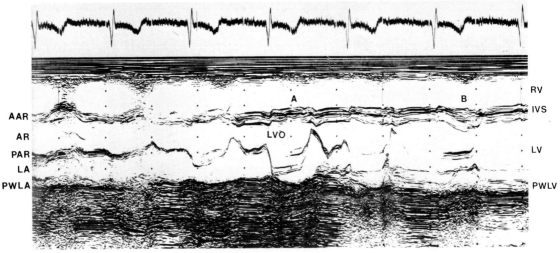

Figure 8–3.   Scan from the aortic root (AR) to the left ventricle (LV). The septum (IVS) is continuous with the anterior wall of the aortic root (AAR). Bordering the left ventricular outflow tract (LVO), the septum moves anteriorly during ventricular systole (a). As the transducer is directed into the body of the left ventricular chamber, the septal motion is reversed, moving posteriorly during systole (b) (PAR = posterior aortic root wall; LA = left atrium; PWLA = posterior wall of the left atrium; RV = right ventricle; PWLV = posterior wall of the left ventricle).

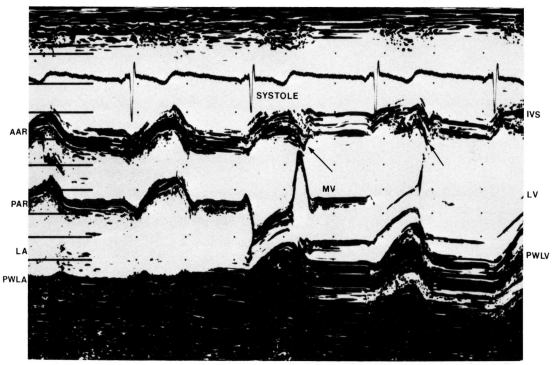

Figure 8-4.   The membranous septum (IVS). Scanning from the left atrium (LA), the septum is contiguous with the anterior wall of the aortic root (AAR). During ventricular systole (following the QRS complex), the membranous septum moves anteriorly with the posterior wall of the left ventricle (PWLV). Immediately following the E point of the mitral valve (MV), it exhibits an abrupt but distinct posteriorly displaced notch (arrow). This septal notch occurs again as the transducer is directed slightly inferiorly from the mitral valve to a position high in the left ventricle (LV) (arrow) (PAR = posterior aortic root wall; PWLA = posterior wall of the left atrium).

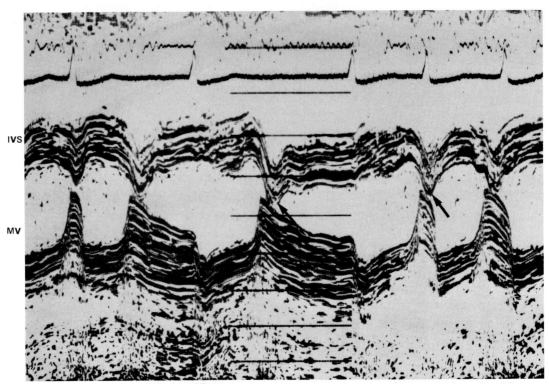

Figure 8–5.   The septal notch in mitral stenosis. The septal notch following the E point of the mitral valve (MV) (arrows) makes the septal motion appear grossly exaggerated (IVS = interventricular septum).

mechanical parameters such as ejection fractions are dependent upon accurately measuring the internal dimension of the left ventricle. It is therefore imperative that the interventricular septum be recorded in the proper position, just beneath the mitral leaflets. This is best accomplished by first placing the transducer in the mitral valve position, in the fourth intercostal space, very close to the sternum, and then directing it inferolaterally off the mitral valve, thereby recording that portion of the septum and posterior left ventricular wall just beneath the mitral apparatus. By slowly angulating the transducer inferiorly and laterally from the fourth intercostal space position (previously described), there is a progressive lessening of mitral valve motion. When this motion has almost completely disappeared and the endocardial surface of the posterior wall of the left ventricle is seen, it should then be possible to record both sides of the septum by "tuning it in" with the TGC (delay) control. Indistinct echoes that appear unattached to the anterior wall of the septum can be eliminated by turning the near gain until the separate band of echoes originating from the right side of the septum is clearly evident. Within the body of the left ventricle, the walls of the septum appear to exhibit an undulating-type motion in place of the zigzag motion at the level of the mitral valve.

The possibility always exists that because of incorrect transducer angulation, septal echoes can be confused with other cardiac echoes, such as those from the chordae tendineae or papillary muscles. In this event, one can return to an easily recognized structure such as the aortic root, which provides an excellent landmark when recording the interventricular septum. After identification of the aortic root has been established (see Chapter 5), the TGC (delay) curve is adjusted to rest on the leading edge of the anterior aortic root. At this point, the reject and/or attenuation is adjusted to eliminate all low-intensity echoes. With gradual angulation of the transducer laterally and inferiorly from the aortic root, the wave form of the posterior aortic root is reduced in amplitude until the mitral leaflets are identified.

From this reference point, the transducer is angled more inferiorly and medially until only the endocardial surface of the posterior left ventricular wall is recognized. No change in the TGC curve is necessary as the anterior aortic root makes its conversion to the interventricular septum (unless the left ventricle is grossly dilated, shifting the septum to a more anterior position relative to the anterior aortic root wall). In addition to having identified the septum, a "sweep" has been executed from the aortic root to the mitral valve and left ventricle (Fig. 8–3). Although this "scanning" technique takes considerable practice, it remains an invaluable method of accurately identifying and recording the interventricular septum. Lastly, it should be emphasized that a successful echocardiographic recording of the interventricular septum requires not only technical expertise but also ultrasonic equipment with sensitive gain controls, so that the septum *can* be "tuned in" individually without affecting echoes from the more distal structures.

SEPTAL THICKNESS

Maximal septal thickness occurs midway between the aortic root and the left ventricular apex.[2] Therefore, septal thickness and movement are best seen just below the mitral valve leaflets, which requires the echo beam to intersect the septum at or near a 90-degree angle on this plane (Fig. 8–6).[3] If the echo beam strikes the septum at a more oblique angle, it may appear falsely thickened. In the normal heart, the thickness of the muscular septum and posterior left ventricular wall are approximately equal, ranging from 0.9 cm to 1.1 cm. The width of the septum varies with systole and diastole. During ventricular systole, the septum thickens by approximately one third and reaches its smallest width in late diastole. The width of the septum is measured at end-diastole, immediately preceding the P wave or at the initial predominant R wave or S wave of the QRS complex of the electrocardiogram, when it is relatively motionless (Fig. 8–2). Septal echoes that are not present continuously throughout an entire cardiac cycle or that appear only during systole or diastole should not be considered true septal echoes. This type of signal is usually the result of suboptimal transducer angulation.

Abnormal thickening of the septum may occur secondarily, as in calcific aortic stenosis with left ventricular myocardial hypertrophy. Both the septum and the posterior ventricular wall are similarly thickened in the concentric forms of myocardial hypertrophy (see Chapter 7). A thick but normally moving septum with normal posterior wall thickness may occur in right ventricular hypertrophy. Finally, there are cases where the septum is grossly thickened by the primary pathologic process known as asymmetric septal hypertrophy (ASH) which may cause left ventricular outflow tract obstruction.[4] A number of echocardiographic features may be seen with this disease.[5] Together with the large, immobile septum, the left ventricular cavity tends to be small and the posterior wall motion sometimes vigorous. An abnormal motion of the anterior mitral valve leaflet usually contributes to the obstruction. The mitral valve appears compressed within the cavity and will strike the septum during initial diastolic opening and may lie against it for most of diastole. During systole, the anterior mitral valve leaflet is displaced anteriorly towards, or even against, the septum. The aortic valve opens normally, but in mid-systole, it often exhibits total or partial closure followed in late diastole by reopening. There will usually be some left atrial enlargement. Figures 8–7 to 8–9 demonstrate some of the various characteristics of ASH. This is also discussed in Chapters 4 and 5.

FACTORS ALTERING SEPTAL MOTION

Variations in transducer angulation can produce changes in septal motion. For instance, an erroneous diagnosis of "paradoxical" septal motion may be made if the echo beam intersects the septum at such a high point on that structure that the mitral valve is seen in its entirety. However, when the echo beam intersects the septum at the level below the mitral valve leaflets and passes through the body of the left ventricle in a plane perpendicular to these structures, its posterior systolic motion will appear fairly constant (Fig. 8–10).

Text continued on page 180

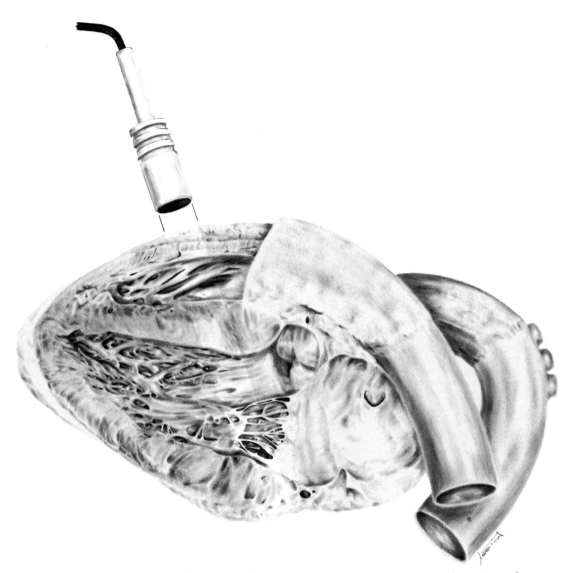

Figure 8–6. The ultrasound beam should intercept the septum approximately at its mid-portion and the posterior left ventricular wall just below the mitral valve.

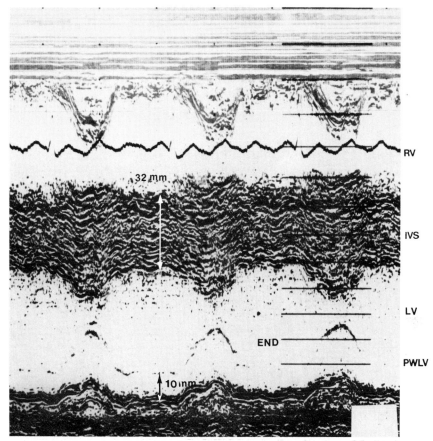

Figure 8–7. The interventricular septum (IVS) and left ventricle (LV) in nonobstructive asymmetric septal hypertrophy (ASH). Asymmetric septal hypertrophy has been defined as an interventricular septum–to–left ventricular posterior wall (PWLV) ratio equal to or exceeding 1.3:1.[4] In this recording, asymmetric septal hypertrophy is demonstrated by a septal thickness of approximately 32 mm, with a normal posterior wall thickness of 10 mm (arrows). The septum–to–posterior wall ratio is 3.2:1. The left ventricular chamber is reduced, and the posterior wall demonstrates good contractility (RV = right ventricle; END = endocardium).

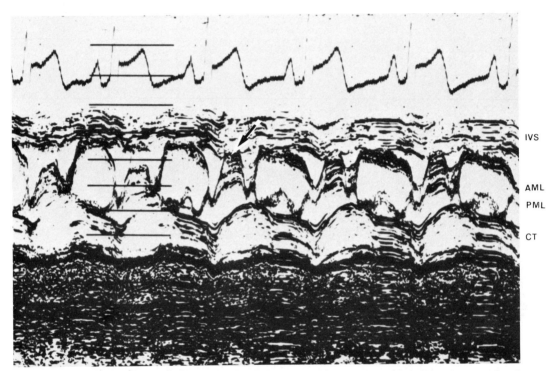

IVS

AML

PML

CT

Figure 8–8.   The mitral valve in obstructive asymmetric septal hypertrophy. The mitral valve anterior leaflet (AML) strikes the septum as it exhibits the characteristic systolic anterior motion (SAM) (arrow). Moving with the anterior mitral leaflet, the posterior mitral leaflet (PML) together with the echoes originating from the chordae tendineae (CT) also demonstrate a pronounced abnormal anterior displacement. In diastole, the excursion of the mitral valve is visibly reduced, and the E-F slope is slowed. The anterior mitral leaflet contacts the septum during most of systole and diastole, consequently participating in obstructing the ventricular outflow tract.

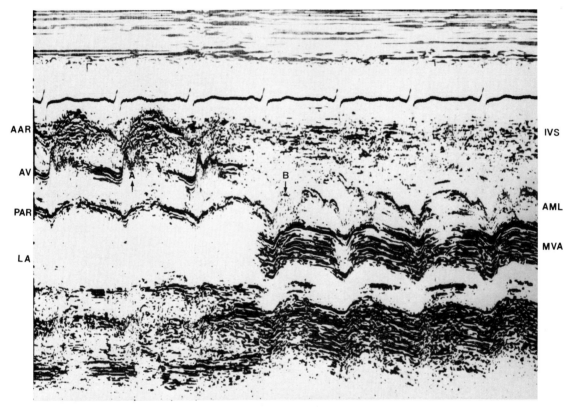

Figure 8–9. Scan from the aortic valve (AV) to the mitral valve in obstructive asymmetric septal hypertrophy. The aortic valve opens normally, but in mid-systole it almost totally closes before moving back to its original systolic position (A). The premature closure of the aortic valve occurs at the same time during the cardiac cycle as the anterior mitral leaflet (AML) exhibits its abnormal systolic motion (B), suggesting that this pattern is secondary to obstruction in the left ventricular outflow tract and is produced by the abnormal movement of the anterior mitral leaflet during systole. Note the grossly thickened mitral valve annulus. The interventricular septum (IVS) is not clearly seen (AAR = anterior wall of the aortic root; PAR = posterior wall of the aortic root; LA = left atrium; MVA = mitral valve annulus).

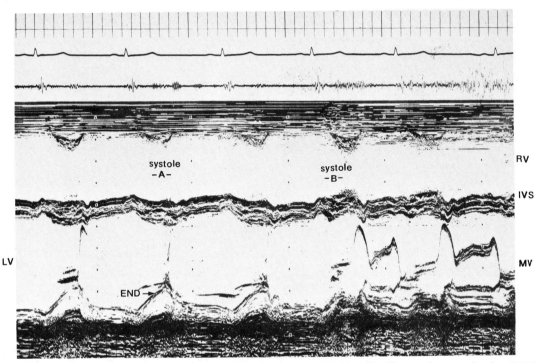

Figure 8–10.   Scan from the left ventricle (LV) just below the mitral leaflets to the mitral valve (MV). In plane A, recorded just below the mitral leaflets, the septum (IVS) exhibits a normal posterior motion during systole. In plane B, with the mitral valve well visualized, its motion is reversed, moving anteriorly in systole. The septal motion in plane B should not be erroneously mistaken for a "paradoxical" septum (RV = right ventricle; END = endocardium [arrow]).

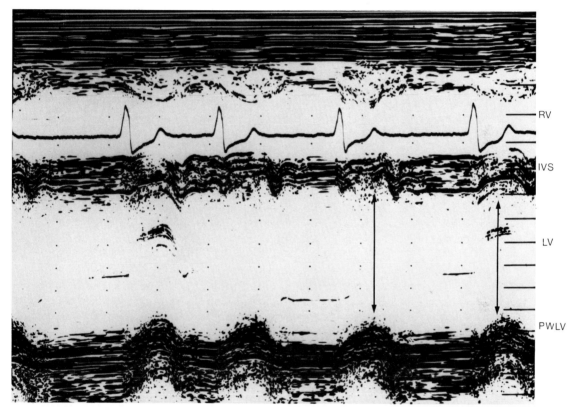

Figure 8–11.   Reversed (type A) septal motion. Secondary to septal infarction, the septum (IVS) exhibits a paradoxical pattern, moving anteriorly during systole in parallel with the posterior wall of the left ventricle (PWLV) (arrows) (RV = right ventricle; LV = left ventricle).

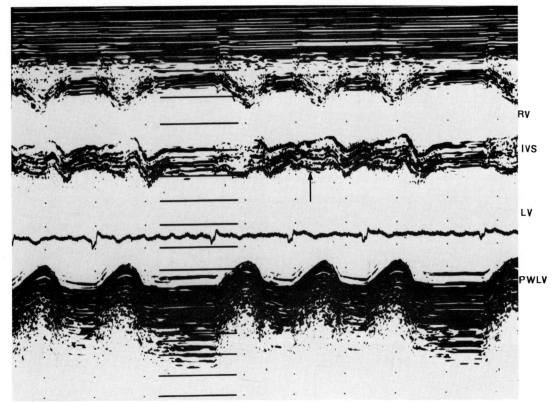

Figure 8–12.   Flattened (type B) septal motion. During systole, the septum (IVS) exhibits practically no movement (arrow) (RV = right ventricle; LV = left ventricle; PWLV = posterior wall of the left ventricle).

Diamond et al.[6] have categorized changes in systolic septal motion in adults as (1) paradoxical, or anterior, motion during systole, resulting in a parallel motion of the interventricular septum and posterior heart wall (Fig. 8–11), and (2) flattened, with relatively little systolic motion (Fig. 8–12). The abnormal paradoxical motion has been designated "Type A" motion and the flattened septal motion, "Type B." Depending upon the underlying cause, any of several mechanisms can produce abnormal septal motion. The most common causes are right ventricular volume overload, a conduction defect, such as left bundle branch block, and infarction of the septum.

Right Ventricular Volume Overload

As mentioned in Chapter 7, volume overloading of the left ventricle increases its stroke volume and results in more vigorous motion of its walls. However, where there is volume overloading of the right ventricle, as

with atrial septal defect or pulmonic or tricuspid insufficiency, the echocardiographic septal motion is usually anterior, away from the left ventricular wall during systole. Meyer et al.[7] have proposed that the paradoxical septal motion is the result of the more anterior position of the right ventricle when it is dilated, with rotation of the left ventricle posteriorly.[8] When an excessive volume of blood is ejected from the right ventricle, the amplitude from the anterior movement of the heart exceeds the posterior motion of the septum and causes the septum to move anteriorly during systole (Fig. 8–13).

Left Bundle Branch Block

The bundle branches are part of the specialized transmission system that distributes the electrical stimulus throughout the ventricular muscle. They are divided into two branches, the right and left bundles, which descend on opposite sides of the in-

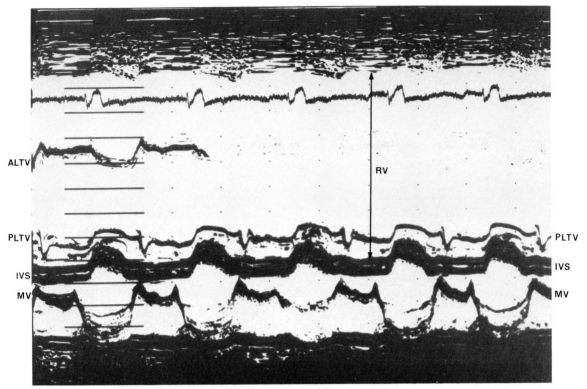

Figure 8–13. The septum in right ventricular volume overload. The right ventricle (RV) is grossly dilated (arrow). Portions of the tricuspid valve posterior leaflet (PLTV) can be seen just anterior to the interventricular septum (IVS). The septal motion is anterior during ventricular systole (ALTV = anterior leaflet of the tricuspid valve; MV = mitral valve).

terventricular septum. When the left branch of the bundle (left bundle branch) or its peripheral branches are blocked, left ventricular activation is delayed, and the sequence of timing in relation to septal contraction is disturbed. Echocardiography has confirmed this supposition by demonstrating a distinctly abnormal septal motion that exhibits an early and abrupt posterior displacement during the pre-ejection period (immediately following the onset of the QRS complex of the electrocardiogram) before the delayed commencement of contraction of the posterior wall of the left ventricle.[9] In many cases of left bundle branch block, the septum will also move in a paradoxical fashion during ejection of blood from the ventricle.

In some cases of calcific aortic stenosis, strong echoes from an immobile septum may be suggestive that it, too, is calcified; this observation is often made in patients with pacemakers, suggesting that septal calcification may be the cause of their heart block.

Myocardial Infarction

Anteroseptal myocardial infarction may also cause paradoxical septal motion.[10] Feigenbaum[11] has pointed out that in the presence of occlusive disease of the left anterior descending coronary artery, there is usually diminished, flat, or paradoxical motion of the interventricular septum (Fig. 8–14). It should be emphasized that to date, the echocardiogram alone is not sufficient in the diagnosis of myocardial infarction. Occasionally, when the infarction is high on the septum, a recording may demonstrate an area of regional akinesis (Fig. 8–15). As the echo beam is angled steadily downward from the mitral valve, special motion will initially be normal, then will diminish or even become paradoxical, and finally may return to normal as the echo beam intersects a plane near the apex. It is also possible to miss an area of septal infarction, especially if it involves the lower third or posterior aspect of the septum.[3] To minimize the possibility of obtaining such false impressions,

Text continued on page 186

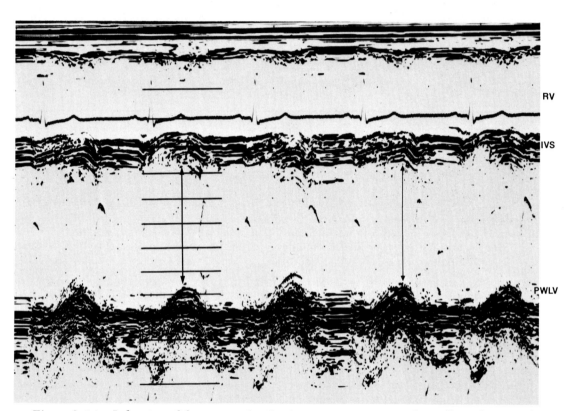

Figure 8–14. Infarction of the septum (IVS). The septum moves paradoxically in the same direction as the posterior wall of the left ventricle (PWLV) during ventricular systole (arrows). The thickening in systole that is seen with normal septal motion is absent. The left ventricular wall shows good contractility (RV = right ventricle).

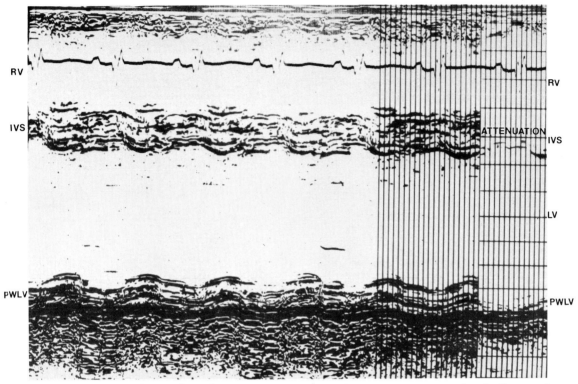

Figure 8-15. Infarction of the septum (IVS). The infarcted septum appears as a band of heavy, distinct parallel echoes. There is a marked decrease in septal motion with diminished posterior left ventricular wall (PWLV) excursion as well (RV = right ventricle; LV = left ventricle).

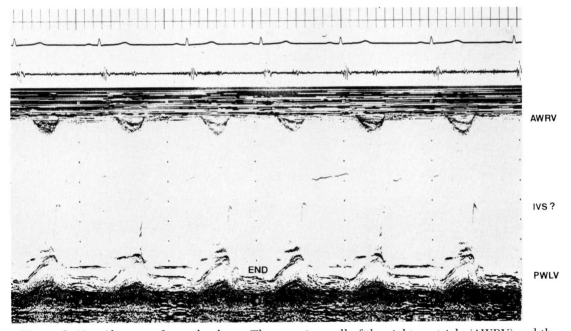

Figure 8-16. Absence of septal echoes. The anterior wall of the right ventricle (AWRV) and the posterior wall of the left ventricle (PWLV) are clearly visualized. The septum (IVS), however, is missing owing to incorrect placement of the TGC (delay) control (see Figure 8-2). Without the septal echoes, it is impossible to obtain a right and left ventricular dimension (END = endocardium).

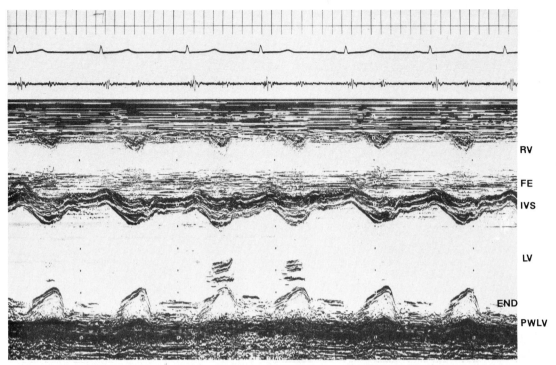

RV

FE

IVS

LV

END

PWLV

Figure 8–17. False right septal (IVS) echoes. The TGC (near gain) curve is erroneously placed at a point between the right ventricle (RV) and the right septal wall. This control should be positioned to rest against the leading edge of the right septal wall (see Figure 8–2). Before septal motion and thickness can be totally assessed, both sides of the septum must be distinct (FE = false echoes; LV = left ventricle; PWLV = posterior wall of the left ventricle; END = endocardium).

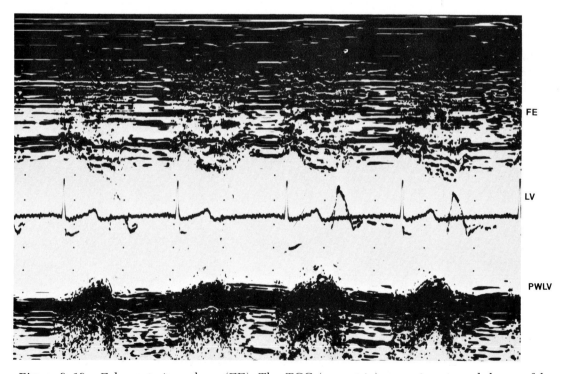

FE

LV

PWLV

Figure 8–18. False anterior echoes (FE). The TGC (near gain) curve is not used; hence, false echoes are allowed to obscure the right ventricle (RV) and the interventricular septum (IVS) (see Figure 8–2) (LV = left ventricle; PWLV = posterior wall of the left ventricle).

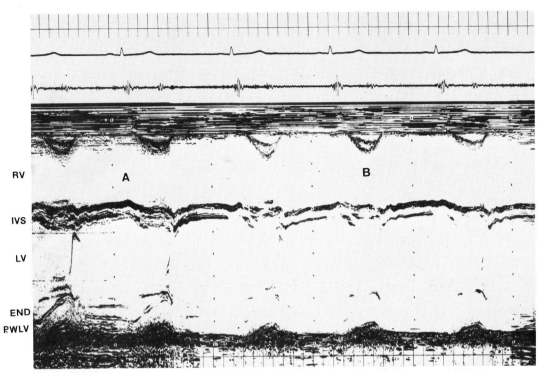

Figure 8–19. The effect of gain control. The area designated A shows correct usage of the overall gain. Both the septum (IVS) and the endocardial (END) surface of the posterior wall of the left ventricle (PWLV) are clearly visualized. The area designated B shows the result of using too little gain and increased reject. There is a loss in the clarity of the septal echoes, and the endocardial surface of the left ventricular wall is absent (RV = right ventricle; LV = left ventricle).

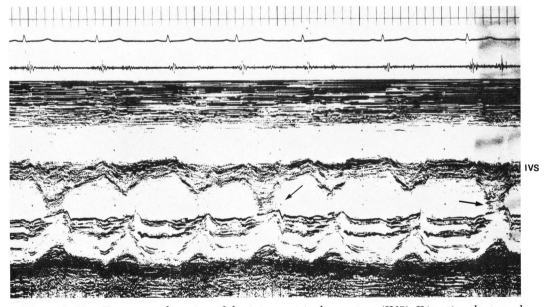

Figure 8–20. Exaggerated motion of the interventricular septum (IVS). Directing the transducer toward the cardiac apex causes an exaggerated septal motion in its posterior direction during systole (arrows). In this tracing, the internal dimension of the left ventricle is difficult to measure accurately.

scans of as much of the septum as possible should be considered routine in every case of coronary disease.[12]

TECHNICAL ERRORS

Figures 8–16 to 8–20 demonstrate some of the common technical errors in recording the interventricular septum.

REFERENCES

1. McDonald IG, Feigenbaum H, and Chang S: Analysis of the left ventricular wall motion by reflected ultrasound: Application to assessment of myocardial function. Circulation 46:14–25, 1972.
2. Roberts WC: Valvular, subvalvular, and supravalvular aortic stenosis: Morphologic features. Cardiovasc Clin 5:104, 1973.
3. Friedewald VE Jr.: Textbook of Echocardiography. Philadelphia, W. B. Saunders Company, 1977.
4. Henry WL, Clark CE, and Epstein SE: Asymmetric septal hypertrophy: Echocardiographic identification of the pathognomonic anatomic abnormality of IHSS. Circulation 47:225–233, 1973.
5. Shah PM, Gramiak R, Adelman G, and Wigle ED: Role of echocardiography in diagnostic and hemodynamic assessment of hypertrophic subaortic stenosis. Circulation 44:891, 1971.
6. Diamond MA, Dillon JC, Haine CL, Chang S, and Feigenbaum H: Echocardiographic features of atrial septal defect. Circulation 43:129, 1971.
7. Meyer RA, Schwartz OC, Benzing G, and Kaplan S: Ventricular septum in right ventricular overload: An echocardiographic study. Am J Cardiol 30:349, 1972.
8. McCullagh W, Covell JW, and Ross J: Left ventricular dilation and diastolic compliance during chronic volume overloading. Circulation 45:943, 1972.
9. McDonald IG: Echocardiographic demonstration of abnormal motion of the interventricular septum in left bundle branch block. Circulation 48:272–280, 1973.
10. Feigenbaum H: Echocardiography. Philadelphia, Lea and Febiger, 1972, p. 201.
11. Jacobs JJ, Feigenbaum H, Corya BC, and Phillips JF: Detection of left ventricular asynergy by echocardiography. Circulation 48:263, 1973.
12. Winters WL Jr., and Chapman R: Variations in ventricular septal motion defined by echocardiography (Abstr). Circulation 48:231, 1973.

Chapter 9

THE RIGHT VENTRICLE

The assessment of the right ventricular chamber is a subject of some controversy among investigators in echocardiography today. This is primarily because there is a wide variance in the angle from which the transducer beam may transverse the diameter of this structure. Because of its anatomical position beneath the sternum, the ultrasound beam is usually able to transverse only a small portion of it (Fig. 9–1).[1] Significant enlargement, however, can be easily seen and recorded.

ANATOMY

The right ventricle is the most anterior of the cardiac chambers and in cross-section appears to have a crescent shape. Its walls are considerably thicker than the walls of the atria but thinner than the left ventricular walls. The wall of the right ventricle is approximately 3 to 4 mm in thickness as compared to the thick muscular walls of the left ventricle, which measure approximately 8 to 16 mm (Fig. 9–1).[2]

The interventricular septum forms the medial and posterior walls of the right ventricle. The anterior and inferior walls are lined by coarse, finger-shaped, muscular projections called papillary muscles, which taper into very thin, strong, white cords, the chordae tendineae. These run from the apices of the papillary muscles to the edges of the tricuspid valve leaflets and maintain tension on the leaflets during ventricular systole.

Functionally, the right ventricle is partitioned into an inflow tract, receiving blood from the right atrium through the tricuspid valve, and an outflow tract, whereby the blood leaves the right ventricle through the pulmonary valve.

ECHOCARDIOGRAPHIC APPEARANCE

A-Mode

On the A-mode, the echoes from the anterior chest wall can be visualized as several spikes clustered together anteriorly, on the extreme left of the oscilloscope. About 0.5 cm to the immediate right of this cluster of signals, a thin band of spikes originating from the anterior surface of the right ventricle can be seen. These signals will not appear as those originating from the anterior chest wall and will have a smaller amplitude of motion, moving anteriorly in systole and posteriorly during diastole. From 0.5 to 2.1 cm posterior to the right ventricular signals, the two spikes representing the right and left edges of the interventricular septum can be seen. These signals have basically the same motion as the right ventricular echoes (Fig. 9–2).

M-Mode

The right ventricular chamber, interventricular septum, and left ventricular chamber are identified simultaneously. Discussions of the interventricular septum and left ventricular chamber are found in Chapters 7 and 8. The echoes originating from the right anterior ventricular myocardium can be seen immediately posterior to the echoes originating from the anterior chest wall. The chest wall and anterior myocardial echoes may merge or, in some instances, may be separated by an echo-free space of variable width (Fig. 9–3). This space can sometimes mimic a small anterior effusion. When this question exists,

Text continued on page 193

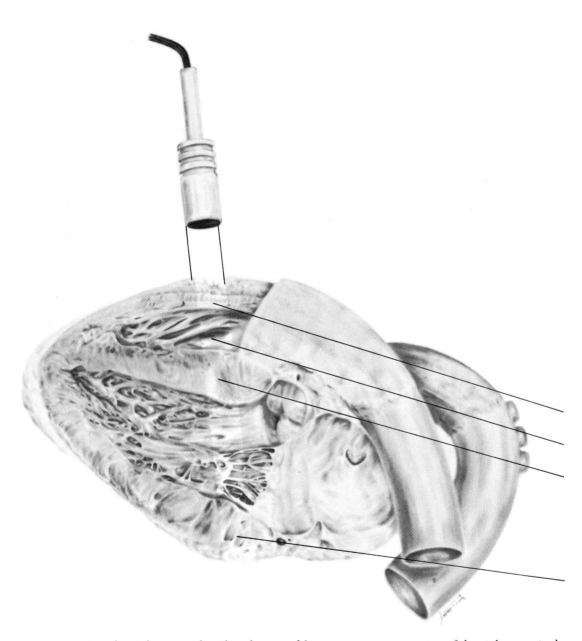

Figure 9–1.   The right ventricle. The ultrasound beam intersects a portion of the right ventricular chamber, the interventricular septum, and the posterior wall of the left ventricle just below the posterior mitral leaflet. Key: AWRV = anterior wall of right ventricle; RVC = right ventricular chamber; IVS = interventricular septum; PWLV = posterior wall of the left ventricle.

AWRV

RVC

IVS

PWLV

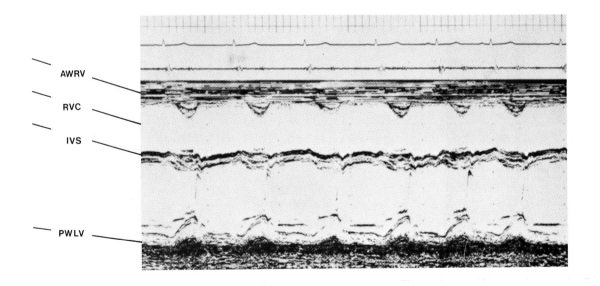

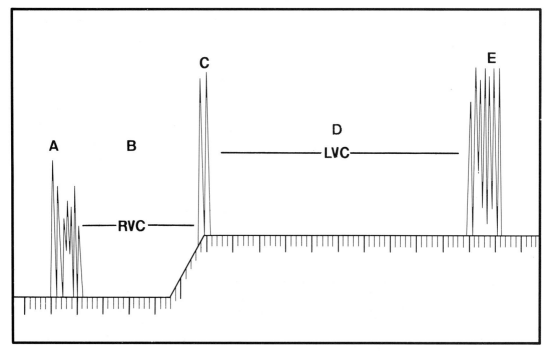

Figure 9–2. In this A-mode schematic representation, the right ventricular chamber (RVC) is depicted as follows: The echoes designated A represent the anterior heart wall and the epicardial surface of the right ventricle. The echo-free space B seen between A and C represents the right ventricular chamber (arrow). C represents the echoes from the interventricular septum. The echo-free space D represents the left ventricular chamber (LVC) (arrow), and the cluster of echoes E arises from the posterior left ventricular wall. Note the placement of the TGC ramp against the leading edge of the septum.

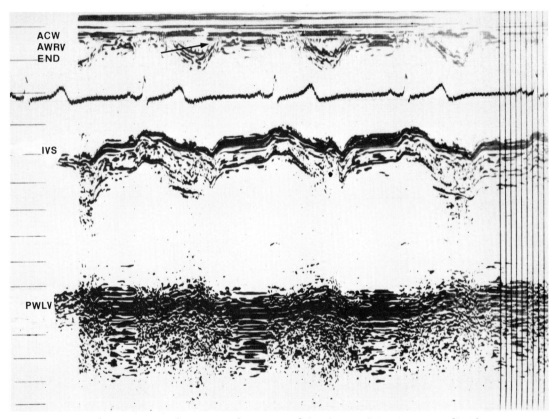

Figure 9–3. The anterior right ventricular myocardium (AWRV) is seen immediately posterior to the anterior chest wall (ACW) and moves in a parallel fashion with the interventricular septum (IVS). The echo-free space between the anterior chest wall and the endocardial (END) surface is a normal finding and is not indicative of pericardial fluid (arrow) (PWLV = posterior wall of the left ventricle).

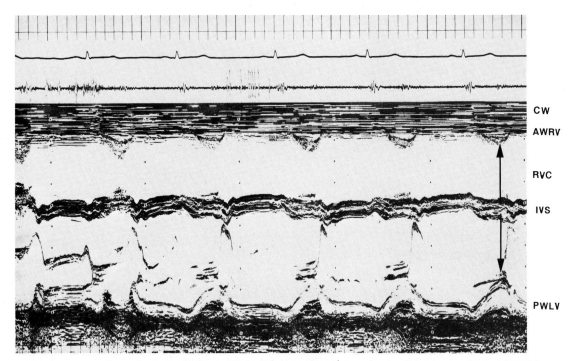

Figure 9-4. The echoes originating from the anterior right ventricular myocardium (AWRV) are clearly seen as a result of proper transducer angulation and adjustment of the "near gain." During ventricular systole, the right ventricular echoes move posteriorly, as opposed to the posterior wall of the left ventricle (PWLV), which moves anteriorly in systole (arrow) (CW = chest wall; RVC = right ventricular chamber; IVS = interventricular septum).

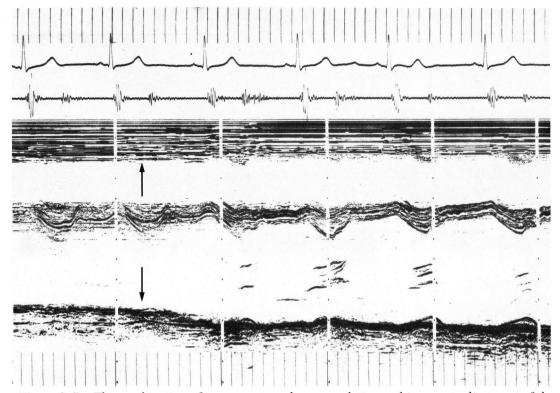

Figure 9-5. The combination of improper transducer angulation and incorrect adjustment of the "near gain" results in the absence of the right ventricular myocardial echoes (arrow). An additional indicator of improper transucer angulation is the flattened appearance and overall loss of left ventricular wall echoes (arrow).

the presence of fluid can usually be ruled out by correct adjustment of the near gain, a slight change in transducer angulation, and the absence of any fluid in the posterior wall of the left ventricle (see Chapter 11).

The right anterior myocardial echoes exhibit a characteristic motion, appearing as a series of "dips" moving posteriorly in systole. This motion is opposite to that of the posterior wall of the left ventricle, which moves anteriorly in systole (Fig. 9–4). With correct transducer angulation and adjustment of instrumentation, the epicardial and endocardial echoes of the right ventricular anterior myocardium will be recognized moving posteriorly toward the interventricular septum during systole. It is not an unusual finding for these echoes to appear as a group of broken or "fuzzy" echoes while maintaining their posterior motion in systole (Figs. 9–4 and 9–5).

RECORDING TECHNIQUE

As with all cardiac echoes, the identification and recording of the right ventricular echoes and chamber is dependent on recognition of their pattern of motion, proper transducer angulation, and precise use of instrumentation. Since the interventricular septum and left ventricular chamber are recorded simultaneously with the right ventricular chamber, the recording technique utilizes the same beam angle as that employed in recording the left ventricular chamber.

After the patient is positioned comfortably, preferably on his left side, a good starting point for transducer placement is in the mitral valve position, in the fourth intercostal space, close to the sternum. It has been our experience that positioning the patient on his left side does not significantly increase the right ventricular dimension.

Following visualization of the mitral valve on the A-mode, slight angulation of the transducer laterally and inferiorly will result in diminished mitral motion. Minute angulation further inferiorly should continue until the systolic excursion of the endocardial echoes of the posterior wall of the left ventricle are seen. The depth or expand control should be adjusted to the point at which the areas of interest are displayed on the oscilloscope. It is extremely difficult to accurately identify the echo patterns on the A-mode if they are grouped too closely together. It may also be necessary to adjust the gain and/or reject controls to eliminate obscuring, excessive echoes. While maintaining clear visualization of the left ventric-

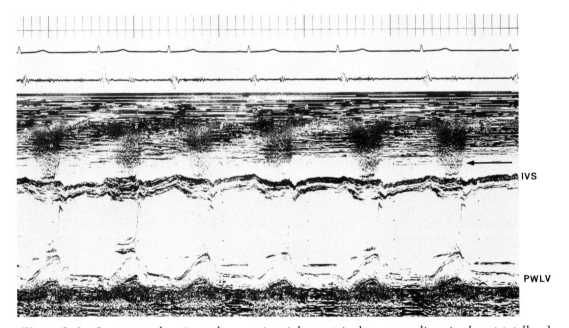

Figure 9–6.   In a normal patient, the anterior right ventricular myocardium is almost totally obscured by excessive echoes as a result of incorrect adjustment of the "near gain" (arrow) (IVS = interventricular septum; PWLV = posterior wall of the left ventricle).

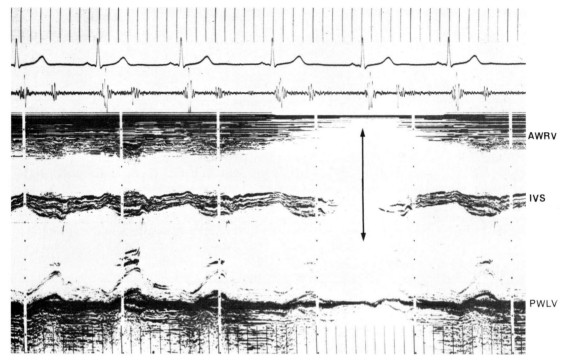

Figure 9–7.   The echoes of the right ventricular myocardium (AWRV) and the septum (IVS) have been "erased" as a result of incorrect adjustment of both the "near gain" and overall "gain" (arrow) (PWLV = posterior wall of the left ventricle).

ular wall, the far gain ramp and/or TGC slope should be adjusted to rest against the leading edge of the interventricular septum, seen moving 3 to 5 cm anterior to the left ventricular wall (Fig. 9–2). When both the left ventricular wall and the septum have been satisfactorily identified, it is then possible to clearly identify the echoes representative of the right ventricular anterior myocardium by simply adjusting the near gain. This near gain control should be slowly turned until the right ventricular wall echoes are seen moving clearly and distinctly on both the A-mode and the M-mode. Proper adjustment of the near gain is somewhat delicate, mainly because the right ventricular anterior myocardium is the first cardiac structure encountered by the ultrasound beam and the ultrasonic energy at this point is considerably increased. Consequently, too much near gain results in excessive right ventricular echoes, and conversely, not enough near gain results in non-visualization of the echoes (Figs. 9–6 and 9–7). In those subjects with left ventricular enlargement, the right ventricular wall is displaced more to a position beneath the sternum, and identifi-

cation of the echoes is facilitated by directing the transducer slightly medially.

MEASUREMENTS

Right Ventricular Dimension

The internal dimension of the right ventricular chamber (RVID) is measured at the onset of the QRS complex of the electrocardiogram from the right ventricular epicardial echo to the leading edge of the anterior wall of the interventricular septum (Fig. 9–8). The normal mean value is 1.5 ± 0.4 cm (range 0.5 to 2.1 cm).[3, 4] Diamond et al.[5] corrected the right ventricular dimension for body surface area and found this to range from 0.3 to 1.1 cm per M[2] (mean 0.7 cm per M[2]). Tajik et al.[4] found that the right ventricular dimension, when corrected for body surface area, varied between 0.8 cm per M[2] for those with a body surface area of 1.0 cm per M[2] or greater, to 1.3 cm per M[2] for those with a body surface area less than 1.0 cm per M[2]. (See Body Surface Area chart in Figure 6–8A.)

The RVID varies considerably among

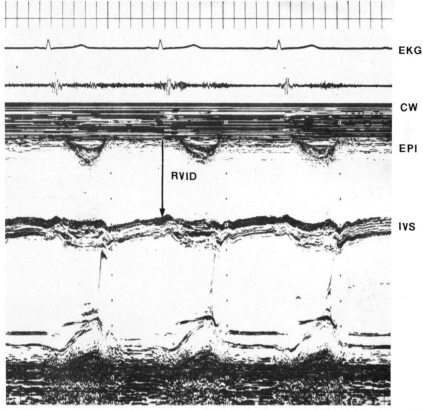

Figure 9–8. The internal dimension of the right ventricle (RVID) is measured from the epicardial edge (EPI) of the right ventricular wall to the right ventricular edge of the interventricular septum (IVS) at the time of the QRS complex of the electrocardiogram (EKG). In this recording, the RVID is minimally enlarged, measuring approximately 2.8 cm (CW = chest wall).

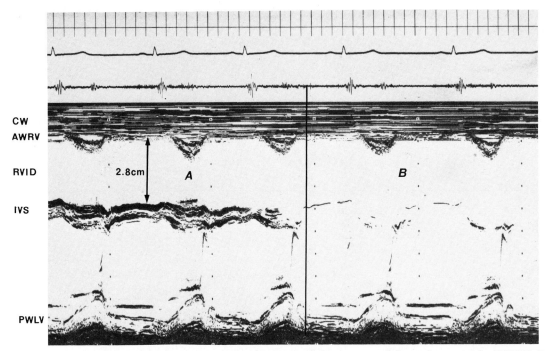

Figure 9–9. Instrumentation in measuring the internal dimension of the right ventricle (RVID). In the section designated A, the RVID can be easily measured (arrow). In section B, however, the "TGC slope" has been incorrectly adjusted to the point at which the septum (IVS) is not seen, making the RVID impossible to measure (CW = chest wall; AWRV = anterior wall of the right ventricle; PWLV = posterior wall of the left ventricle).

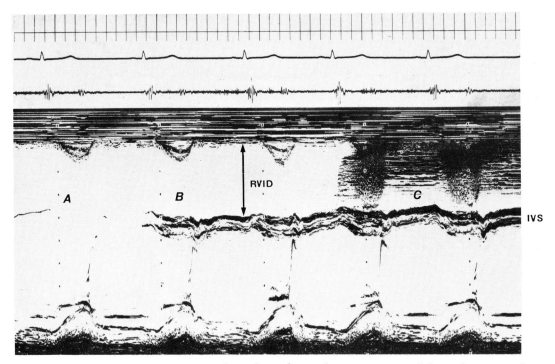

Figure 9–10. Features necessary in the echocardiographic assessment of the right ventricular internal dimension. In section A, the absence of the interventricular septum (IVS) prevents assessment of the RVID. In section B, the necessary right ventricular and septal echoes are present (arrow). The excessive, strong echoes due to incorrect adjustment of the "near gain" in section C prevent accurate measurement of the RVID.

196

normal persons as a result of cardiac rotation, changes in transducer angulation, and in some subjects by respiration.[6] However, by requiring the simultaneous recording of both the interventricular septal and left ventricular wall echoes, the amount of variability is markedly reduced. As a result, the measurements should be more reproducible in multiple or serial examinations of the same patient (Fig. 9–9).

In summary, the three most important factors in the echocardiographic assessment of the RVID are: (1) a good recording of the anterior (right ventricular) edge of the interventricular septum; (2) the elimination of excessive intracavitary echoes between the right ventricular wall and the septum through instrumentation; and (3) determination of the exact motion pattern of the echoes representative of the right ventricular wall. Keeping these three factors in mind will eliminate considerable confusion when

attempting to estimate the internal dimension of the right ventricle (Fig. 9–10).

Right Ventricular Wall Thickness

The thickness of the anterior wall of the right ventricle is sometimes difficult to measure, usually because its anterior border is not easily discernible from the chest wall echoes. There are instances, however, when both the epicardial and endocardial surfaces can be clearly seen (Fig. 9–11). In a study performed on 200 infants, Hagan and associates found the anterior wall thickness in end-diastole to range from 2.0 to 4.7 mm, with a mean range of 3.0 mm. The end-systolic thickness ranged from 3.3 to 7.3 mm, with a mean range of 5.0 mm.[7] Epstein et al. found that the width of the anterior wall increases by only about 0.5 mm from age 6 months to 18

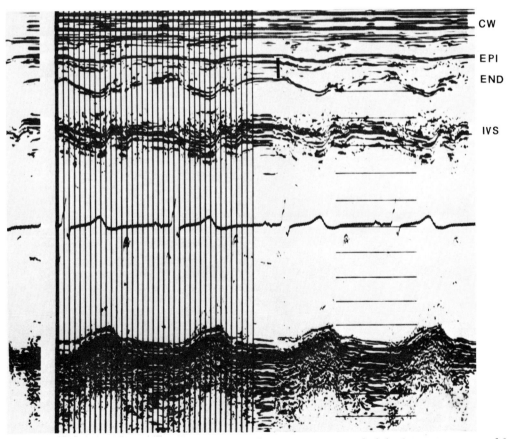

CW

EPI
END

IVS

Figure 9–11.   Right ventricular wall thickness. The anterior myocardial thickness is measured from the epicardial (EPI) to the endocardial (END) surface (arrow). The echo-free space between the chest wall (CW) and the anterior myocardium is representative of subcutaneous tissue and does not demonstrate evidence of a pericardial effusion (IVS = interventricular septum).

years.[8] To date, studies concerning anterior wall thickness have been mostly limited to newborns.

Right Ventricular Outflow Tract

In determining the size of the right ventricular outflow tract, the ratio concept has been employed, comparing the size of the left atrium (LA) to the size of the right ventricular outflow (RVO) tract. This ratio (RVO/LA) is 1.5 in normals.[9] On the echocardiographic recording, the right ventricular outflow tract is seen as an echo-free space anterior to the aortic root (Fig. 9–12).

ASSOCIATED FINDINGS

In patients with atrial septal defects, the right ventricle puts out two to three times the amount of blood as the left; thus, a characteristic echocardiographic finding in these cases is an increased right ventricular internal dimension. An additional echocardiographic feature in these subjects is an abnormal (paradoxical) motion of the interventricular septum (Figs. 9–13 and 9–14).[10, 11] Similar echocardiographic findings have been noted in other conditions that, as in atrial septal defect, also lead to diastolic volume overload of the right ventricle. These conditions include tricuspid insufficiency,[5] partial anomalous pulmonary venous connection with and without associated atrial septal defect,[4] and total anomalous pulmonary venous drainage.[12]

Right ventricular dilatation is often present secondary to mitral valve disease and left ventricular failure (Fig. 9–15).[13]

In cases where there is only a suspicion of right ventricular dilatation, a greater portion of the right ventricular chamber can be visualized by scanning from the left ventricular chamber to the mitral valve and aortic root. This technique is particularly helpful when the heart is rotated and brings a larger portion of the chamber into the path of the

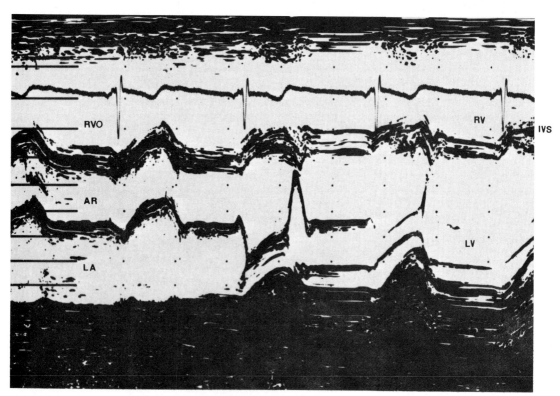

Figure 9–12. The right ventricular outflow tract. In this recording, the transducer has scanned from the aortic root (AR) and the right ventricular outflow tract (RVO), seen anteriorly, to the body of the right ventricle (RV) and left ventricle (LV) (LA = left atrium; IVS = interventricular septum).

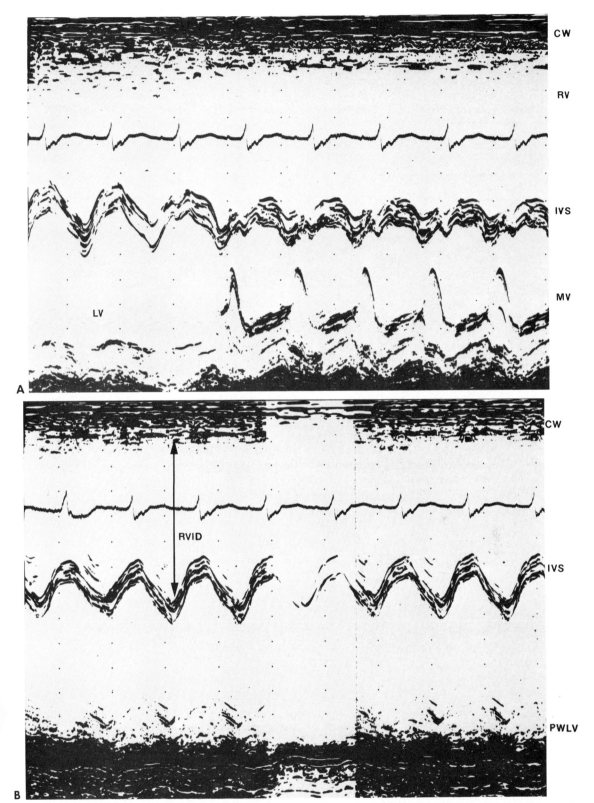

Figure 9–13. (A) Interatrial septal defect. Scanning from the body of the left ventricle to the mitral valve (MV), the septum (IVS) exhibits an exaggerated paradoxical motion. (B) Echocardiogram of the same patient, showing severe right ventricular enlargement (approximately 6.0 cm) and paradoxical septal motion. This patient had a large left to right shunt and recent heart failure (CW = chest wall; IVS = interventricular septum; PWLV = posterior wall of the left ventricle; RVID = right ventricular internal dimension).

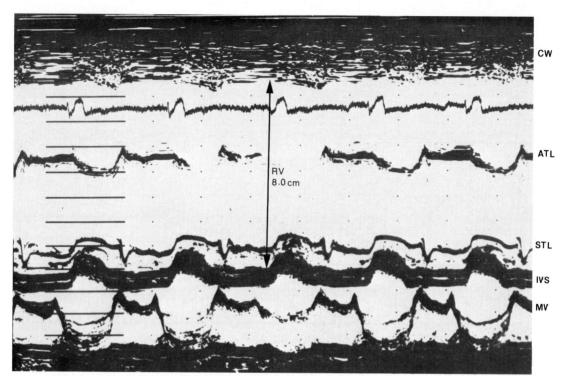

Figure 9–14. Right ventricular dilatation in atrial septal secundum defect. In this recording, the right ventricle is grossly enlarged, measuring approximately 8.0 cm (arrow). In the presence of right ventricular volume overload, the septum (IVS) shows paradoxical motion. Echoes originating from the anterior (ATL) and septal (STL) tricuspid leaflets are also seen. The mitral valve (MV) shows evidence of systolic prolapse (CW = chest wall).

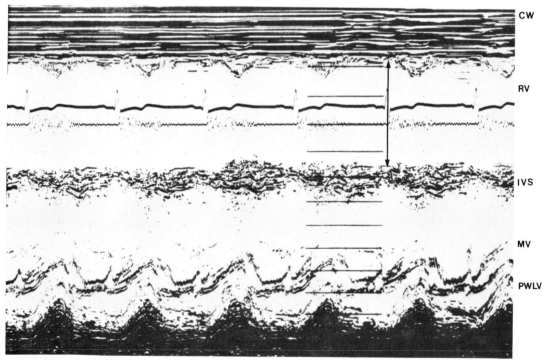

Figure 9–15. The dilated right ventricle in left ventricular failure. In this recording, the right ventricle (RV) measures approximately 4.0 cm. The gross fluttering of the mitral valve (MV) indicates aortic regurgitation. The left ventricle is also dilated (CW = chest wall; IVS = interventricular septum; PWLV = posterior wall of the left ventricle).

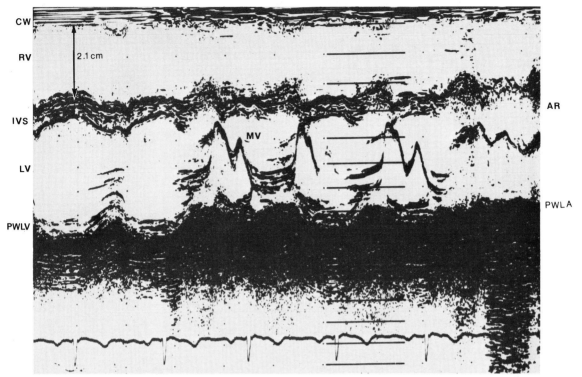

Figure 9–16. This scan from the left ventricle (LV) and right ventricle (RV) to the mitral valve (MV) and aortic root (AR) shows no dilatation of the right ventricular chamber, which measures approximately 2.1 cm. The mitral valve echo indicates systolic prolapse (CW = chest wall; IVS = interventricular septum; PWLV = posterior wall of the left ventricle; PWLA = posterior wall of the left atrium).

ultrasound beam (Fig. 9–16). In the event that the right ventricle is markedly enlarged, as in right ventricular volume overload, the "sweeping" technique is also useful in the assessment of septal motion. If there is a paradoxical motion of the septum, it will be seen in the presence of the mitral valve and will persist as the transducer beam is directed beneath the mitral leaflets into the body of the left ventricular chamber.

REFERENCES

1. Feigenbaum H, Zaky A, and Nasser WK: Use of ultrasound to measure left ventricular stroke volume. Circulation 35:1092, 1967.
2. Hurst JW, and Logue RB (eds.): *The Heart.* New York, McGraw-Hill Book Company, 1970.
3. Popp RL, Wolfe SB, Hirata T, and Feigenbaum H: Estimation of right and left ventricular size by ultrasound: A study of the echoes from the interventricular septum. Am J Cardiol 24:523–530, 1969.
4. Tajik AJ, Gau GT, Ritter DG, and Schattenberg TT: Echocardiographic pattern of right ventricular diastolic volume overload in children. Circulation 46:36–43, 1972.
5. Diamond MA, Dillon JC, Haine CL, Chang S, and Feigenbaum H: Echocardiographic features of atrial septal defect. Circulation 43:129–135, 1971.
6. Goldberg SJ, Allen HD, and Sahn DJ: *Pediatric and Adolescent Echocardiography.* Chicago, Year Book Medical Publishers, Inc., 1975.
7. Hagan AD, Deely WJ, Sahn D, and Friedman WF: Echocardiographic criteria for normal newborn infants. Circulation 48:1221–1226, 1973.
8. Epstein ML, Goldberg SJ, Allen HD, Konecke L, and Wood J: Great vessel, cardiac chamber, and wall growth patterns in normal children. Circulation 51:1124–1129, 1975.
9. Chung KJ, Nanda NC, Manning JA, and Gramiak R: Echocardiographic findings in tetralogy of Fallot (Abstr). Am J Cardiol 31:126, 1973.
10. McCullagh WH, Covell JW, and Ross J Jr.: Left ventricular dilatation and diastolic compliance changes during chronic volume overloading. Circulation 45:943, 1972.
11. Meyer RA, Schwartz DC, Benzing G, and Kaplan S: Ventricular septum in right ventricular volume overload: An echocardiographic study. Am J Cardiol 30:349, 1972.
12. Tajik AJ, Gau GT, and Schattenberg TT: Echocardiogram in total anomalous pulmonary venous drainage: Report of case. Mayo Clin Proc 47:247–250, 1972.
13. Friedewald, VE Jr.: *Textbook of Echocardiography.* Philadelphia, W. B. Saunders Company, 1977.

Chapter 10

THE TRICUSPID AND PULMONIC VALVES

Recording the complete motion of both the tricuspid and pulmonic valves in adult echocardiography can be somewhat difficult owing to the anatomical position of both of these valves behind the sternum. The tricuspid valve, however, is easily recorded when the valve itself is diseased or in the presence of right ventricular dilatation, and the pulmonic valve is usually prominent and easily recorded in the presence of pulmonary hypertension. In either event, recording of these valves may be useful in an echocardiographic diagnosis.

TRICUSPID VALVE

Anatomy

The tricuspid orifice lies medially, slightly inferiorly, and anterior to the mitral orifice. In relation to the pulmonic valve, it lies posteriorly, medially, and inferiorly.

While differences exist, the tricuspid valve, like its mitral counterpart, is an atrioventricular valve. Its components include valve leaflets, an orifice ring (larger than that of the mitral valve), chordae tendineae, and papillary muscles. The three tricuspid leaflets, anterior, posterior, and septal (medial), differ from the mitral leaflets in that they are thinner and more transparent. The anterior leaflet is the longest from its attachment at the annulus to its free surface. The anterior and posterior leaflets, the latter being smallest of the three, attach to the annulus, while the medial leaflet attaches both to the membranous septum and the muscular portion of the septum that forms

202

the posterior wall of the right ventricle. Because of the lower pressures of the right side of the heart, the tricuspid valve is not subjected to the strain of its bicuspid counterpart, the mitral valve.[1]

Echocardiographic Appearance

A-Mode

On the A-mode, the tricuspid valve exhibits the same whiplike motion as the mitral valve. The major distinction lies in its location to the left, anterior to the echoes reflected from the aortic root. The distance from the tricuspid leaflet to the anterior chest wall is approximately 3.5 cm, and from the mitral leaflet, it is approximately 5.8 cm. In contrast to the subtle motion of the aortic root or the interventricular septum, the tricuspid valve has a far greater range of anterior-posterior motion. The tall, rapidly moving spike representing the anterior leaflet of the tricuspid valve has a range of anterior-posterior motion of approximately 2.5 to 4.0 cm.

The spike representing the posterior leaflet of the tricuspid valve exhibits the same whiplike motion as the anterior leaflet, although to a smaller degree and with less amplitude since this leaflet is anatomically smaller. As in the motion of the mitral valve, the anterior and posterior leaflets of the tricuspid valve move in opposition to each other. In the normal adult, the spike originating from the anterior tricuspid leaflet is 2 to 3 cm in amplitude, with the posterior and medial leaflet spikes being closer to 2 cm.

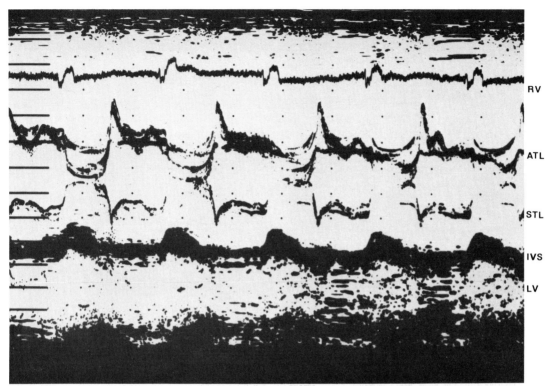

Figure 10–1.   The normal tricuspid valve. In the presence of right ventricular enlargement, both the anterior (ATL) and the septal (STL) tricuspid leaflets are recorded. The motion of the tricuspid valve is similar to that of the normal mitral valve, showing a typical "M" configuration during diastole. The motion of the interventricular septum (IVS) is paradoxical (RV = right ventricle; LV = left ventricle).

In systole, the three signals representative of the tricuspid valve merge into a single cluster of signals.

M-Mode

The M-mode echocardiographic appearance of the anterior leaflet of the tricuspid valve, like that of the mitral valve, can be described as having either an "M" configuration or a "dog-eared" configuration. This distinctive appearance, with the two peaks representative of anterior motion during each cardiac cycle, can be found consistently in normal individuals (Fig. 10–1). Again, the major difference in the echocardiographic appearance of the two valves is that the tricuspid valve lies anterior to the position of the mitral valve (Fig. 10–2).

Recording Technique

Using the aortic valve as a landmark, the tricuspid valve may be detected by placing the transducer at the fourth intercostal space at the left sternal border and tilting it 30 to 45 degrees medially. If the third intercostal space is used, the transducer should be angulated medially and slightly inferiorly from the left sternal border. Because the echoes originating from the anterior heart are stronger and tend to appear as a single grouping, instrumentation adjustment is particularly important when looking for the tricuspid valve. The depth and/or expand controls should be adjusted, extending the echo trace to where the anterior structures are individually recognized. Then, by reducing the near gain, the strong mass of anterior echoes may be lessened, allowing visualization of the tricuspid valve.

Since the echocardiographic configuration of the tricuspid valve is identical to that of the mitral valve, there may be some confusion as to which valve is being recorded. This can be avoided, however, by sweeping from the tricuspid valve to the aortic root and mitral valve. This technique not only guarantees the correct identification of each

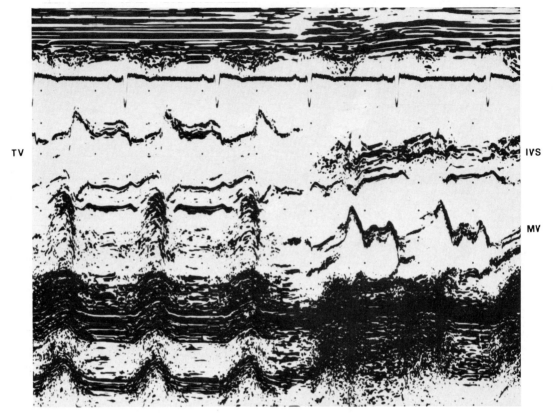

Figure 10–2. The tricuspid valve in relation to the mitral valve. In this scan, the normal anterior position of the tricuspid valve (TV) to the mitral valve (MV) is seen (IVS = interventricular septum).

valve but may also rule out specific pathologies, such as congenital malformations.

To execute the mitral-aortic-tricuspid sweep properly, it is necessary to have a firm understanding of the interrelationships of the intracardiac structures involved.

Located adjacent to each other on the left side of the heart, the mitral and aortic valves are separated only by the membranous septum. Inferiorly, this structure forms the anterior cusp of the mitral valve, and superiorly, it forms the left coronary cusp of the aortic valve. In contrast, the demarcation between the muscular and the membranous septum on the right side of the heart is quite distinct. The posterior cusp of the tricuspid valve is attached to the membranous septum, and the anterior and medial cusps of the tricuspid valve are attached to the base of the right ventricle. This continuity of the anterior mitral leaflet with the posterior aortic root and of the posterior tricuspid leaflet with the anterior aortic root is demonstrated

in the sweep from one structure to another (Fig. 10–3).

In patients with right ventricular dilatation, the tricuspid valve is usually easily recognized and recorded (Fig. 10–1). This is probably due to the fact that the heart rotates to a point where the tricuspid valve is displaced from its normal position behind the sternum into a more lateral position. In these subjects, the tricuspid and mitral valves can often be recorded simultaneously (Figs. 10–4 and 10–5).

Associated Abnormalities of the Tricuspid Valve

Tricuspid Stenosis

The tricuspid valve can usually be well visualized in the presence of severe mitral stenosis because of right ventricular enlargement. In these cases, the two valves

Text continued on page 210

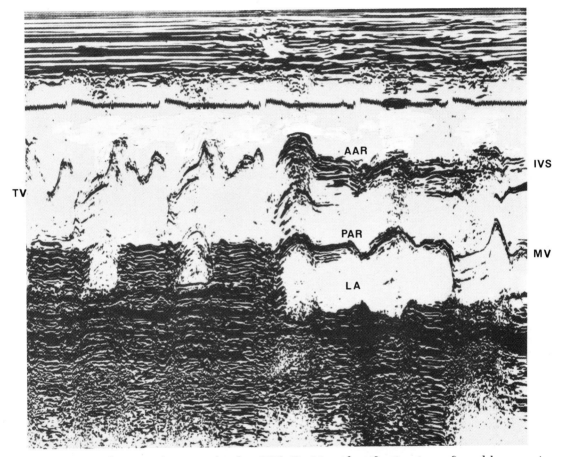

Figure 10–3.   The normal tricuspid valve (TV). Positive identification is confirmed by scanning from the tricuspid valve to the aortic root, with which the tricuspid is continuous, to the anterior aortic root (AAR). The anterior leaflet of the mitral valve (MV) is continuous with the posterior wall of the aortic root (PAR) (LA = left atrium; IVS = interventricular septum).

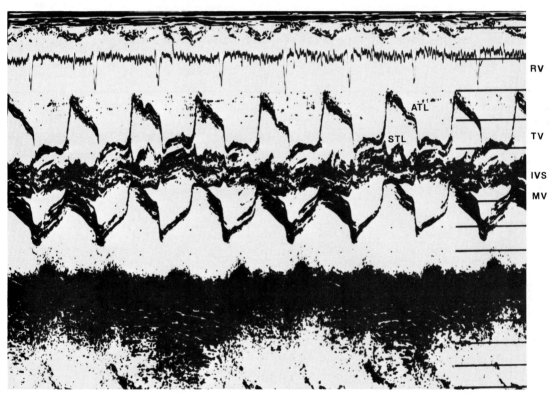

Figure 10–4. Simultaneous recording of the tricuspid valve (TV) and the mitral valve (MV). Both the anterior tricuspid (ATL) and the septal (STL) leaflets are seen. The mitral valve appears slightly thickened and is mildly stenotic. The right ventricle (RV) is dilated (IVS = interventricular septum).

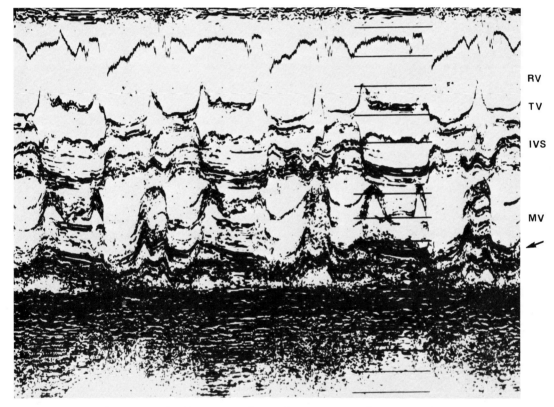

Figure 10–5.   The tricuspid valve (TV) and mitral valve (MV). The tricuspid valve is easily record-ed within a grossly dilated right ventricle (RV). The mitral valve is thickened and is suggestive of holo-systolic prolapse. The increased echoes behind it bear some resemblance to a left atrial myxoma (ar-row) (IVS = interventricular septum).

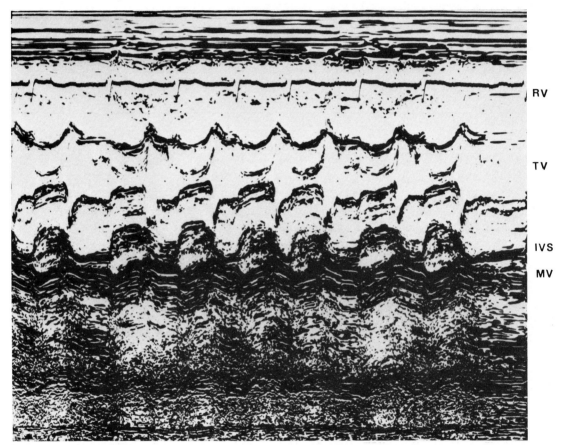

RV

TV

IVS

MV

Figure 10–6.   The tricuspid valve (TV) in mitral stenosis. Visualization of the mitral valve (MV) is difficult owing to marked thickening (RV = right ventricle; IVS = interventricular septum).

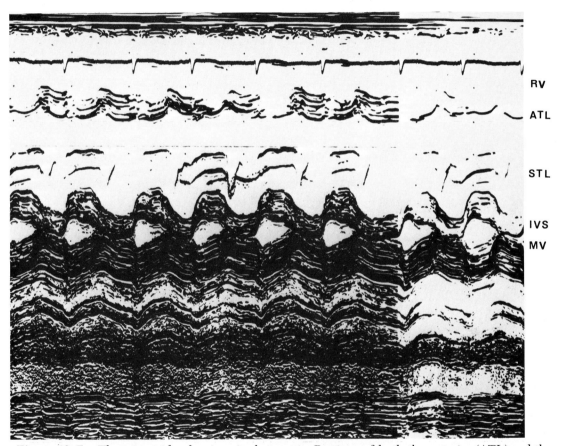

RV

ATL

STL

IVS

MV

Figure 10-7.   The tricuspid valve in mitral stenosis. Portions of both the anterior (ATL) and the septal (STL) tricuspid leaflets are seen. The echoes have been dampened owing to excessive mitral valve (MV) thickness secondary to severe mitral stenosis (RV = right ventricle; IVS = interventricular septum).

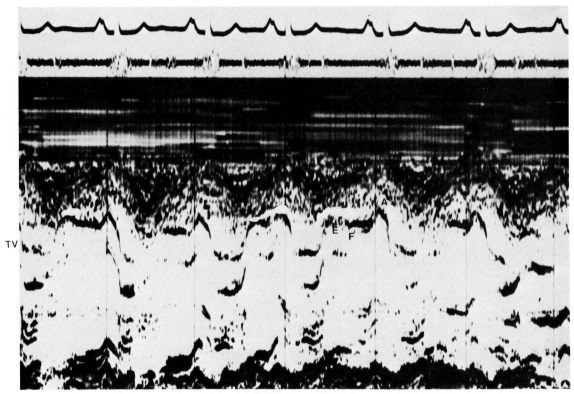

Figure 10–8.   Tricuspid stenosis. The E-F slope is markedly reduced in the presence of stenosis. The A point is preserved (TV = tricuspid valve).

may be recorded simultaneously, permitting good visualization of the tricuspid motion (Figs. 10–6 and 10–7). The echocardiographic diagnosis of tricuspid stenosis is not well established, but as in mitral stenosis, the diastolic descent (E-F) slope is markedly reduced to under 35 mm/sec (Fig. 10–8).[2] One should always be alerted to the possibility of false positives of tricuspid stenosis, especially in patients who do not show evidence of this condition. Technical errors such as improper transducer angulation can easily produce a "pseudo" reduced tricuspid E-F slope. A reduced E-F slope may also be seen in the presence of pulmonary hypertension or a reduction in right ventricular compliance. Just as decreased left ventricular compliance produces a reduced E-F mitral closure, decreased right ventricular compliance produces a reduced E-F tricuspid closure.[3, 4]

Tricuspid Valve Fluttering

Diastolic fluttering of the tricuspid valve may be the result of pulmonic regurgitation

when the regurgitant jet strikes it during diastole (Fig. 10–9).[5] Diastolic tricuspid fluttering has also been observed as a result of increased flow in the presence of an atrial septal defect (Fig. 10–10),[6] transposition of the great vessels,[7] and congenital communication from the left ventricle to the right atrium.[8]

Tricuspid Regurgitation

Although an increased amplitude has been observed in the echocardiographic diagnosis of tricuspid regurgitation, to date there are few echocardiographic criteria for this abnormality.[2] Tricuspid prolapse has been associated with regurgitation.[9] This has been described as a systolic sagging displacement of the valve similar to that observed in patients with prolapsing mitral valves (Fig. 10–11).[8] However, the reliability of a diagnosis of tricuspid prolapse remains uncertain, and considerable additional echocardiographic data will be required before the diagnosis of systolic prolapse can be documented by echocardiography.

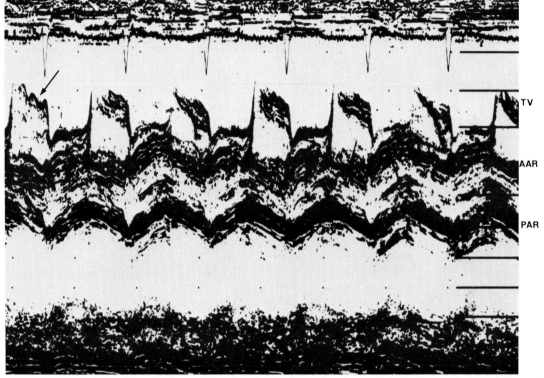

Figure 10–9. Diastolic fluttering of the tricuspid valve (TV). Fluttering of the anterior leaflet (ATL) (arrow) occurs secondary to pulmonary incompetence. The anterior tricuspid leaflet is recorded along with the anterior wall of the aortic root (AAR) (PAR = posterior wall of the aortic root).

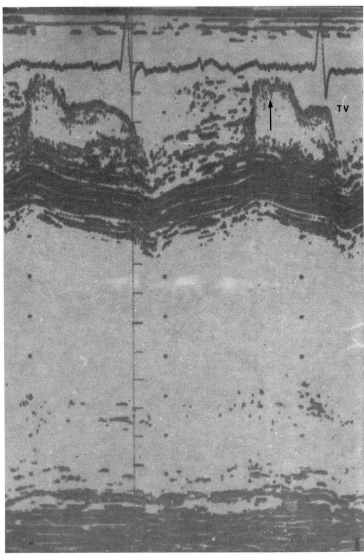

Figure 10–10.   The tricuspid valve in atrial septal defect. Fluttering of the tricuspid valve (TV) (arrow) during diastole is seen secondary to a large atrial septal defect.

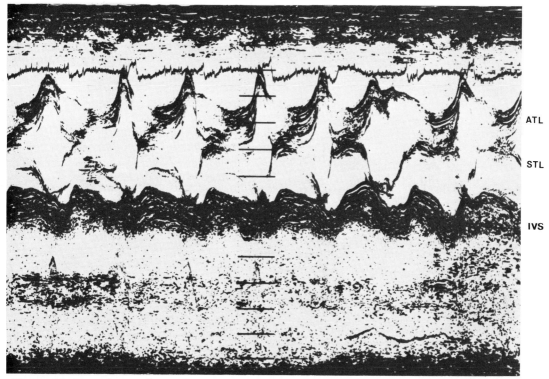

ATL

STL

IVS

Figure 10-11.   Abnormal systolic motion associated with regurgitation. During systole, the tricuspid leaflets exhibit a marked sagging motion, typical of the echocardiographic features of a holosystolic mitral valve prolapse. The anterior leaflet (ATL) shows a large range of excursion, and the valve itself appears abnormally prominent (STL = septal tricuspid leaflet; IVS = interventricular septum).

Ebstein's Malformation

Ebstein's anomaly is a congenital abnormality in which the tricuspid valve is abnormally attached to the right ventricular myocardium with a resultant downward displacement into the right ventricular chamber. The functioning valvular tissue is usually composed of the anterior leaflet alone. The valve leaflet appears large, with a prominent excursion, and may merge with the anterior myocardial and chest wall echoes.[3, 4, 10, 11] A specific characteristic feature for the diagnosis of Ebstein's anomaly is a delay in closure of the tricuspid valve as compared to closure of the mitral valve of 0.04 to 0.10 sec.[10, 12]

THE PULMONIC VALVE

Anatomy

The orifice of the pulmonic valve lies at the junction of the pulmonary artery and the right ventricle, anterior and superior to, and slightly left of, the aortic valve. Like the aortic valve, the pulmonic valve is a semilunar structure and is composed of three cusps, the anterior, right, and left. Although similar in character, the pulmonic cusps are thinner than the aortic cusps and are subjected to the lower pressures of the right heart. The mean pulmonary artery systolic pressure is approximately 24 mm Hg.[1]

When the right ventricle contracts, the pulmonic valve opens, and blood is forced into the pulmonary artery. When the chamber relaxes, the valve closes to prevent a backflow of the blood that has been directed to the lungs.

Echocardiographic Appearance

A-Mode

On the A-mode, the pulmonary artery shows the same characteristic parallel-moving double echoes as the aortic root, appearing as two distinct echo signals of equal amplitude with relatively little motion. Moving rapidly between the walls of the pulmonary artery, the echoes originating from the pulmonic valve cusps are seen as three separate and rather delicate signals.

The pulmonic valve is located to the extreme left, anterior and superior to the aortic root.

M-Mode

On the M-mode, the margins of the pulmonary artery are seen as two parallel echoes, approximately 2 to 4 cm apart and located anterior to the aortic root. Depending on transducer angulation, the aortic root may not be seen in the same view as the pulmonary artery.

In optimal recordings, the complete pattern of the pulmonic valve resembles the aortic valve and will be seen moving between the walls of the pulmonary artery (Fig. 10–12). Because of the anatomical position of the valve and its plane of motion relative to the ultrasound beam, the echocardiogram usually records only the left pulmonic cusp. In relation to the electrocardiogram, the various motions of the left pulmonic cusp have been designated by the letters A, B, C, D, E, and F (Fig. 10–13).[13] Immediately following the P wave of the electrocardiogram, the left cusp exhibits a short posterior motion, termed the "A" wave. This short pre-systolic motion reflects the effect of atrial contraction. In a study performed by Weyman et al.,[14] the normal "A" wave deflection averaged 3.7 mm (with a range of 2 to 7 mm). After the QRS complex, the left cusp from point B rapidly moves to a fully open position at a rate of less than 300 mm per sec (B-C segment).[3, 15] During systole, when the leaflet is in the fully open position (C-D), portions of the echoes may be lost in the dense mass of echoes behind the pulmonary artery. At the end of the systole, the valve moves to its closed diastolic position (D-E segment) with a forward and inferior motion. It then moves slowly posteriorly until late diastole (E-F segment). Weyman et al. have determined the average normal pulmonic valve E-F slope to be 36.9 ± 25.4 mm per sec with a wide range, from 6 to 115 mm per sec.[14]

Recording Technique

Two standard techniques for examining the pulmonic valve have been described. In the first approach, described by Gra-

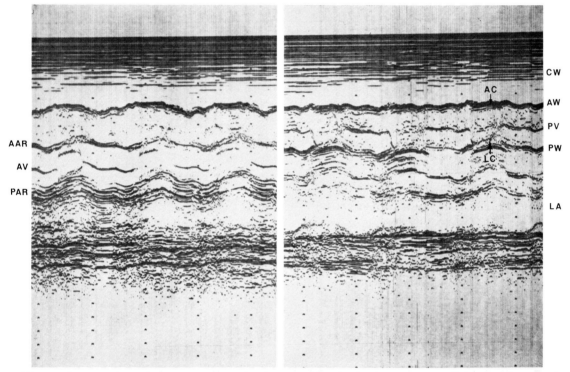

Figure 10–12. The pulmonary artery and pulmonic valve (PV). The anterior wall (AW) of the vessel lies just posterior to the chest wall (CW). In this recording, both the anterior (AC) and left (LC) valve cusps are seen. To the left of the recording, the walls of the aortic root (AAR, PAR) and aortic valve (AV) are seen immediately beneath the posterior wall of the pulmonary artery (PW) (LA = left atrium).

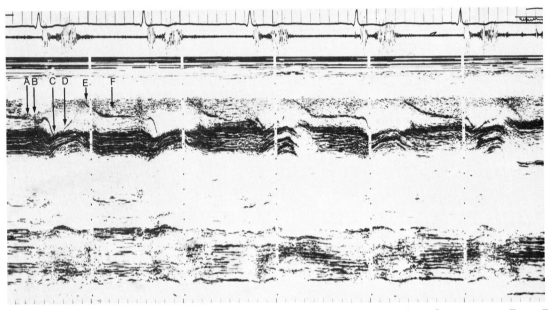

Figure 10–13.   The left pulmonic cusp. The A wave reflects the effect of atrial contraction. Point B represents the position of the leaflet at the onset of ventricular ejection; B-C is the rapid systolic opening of the leaflet. Valve closure occurs at the D point, and E-F represents closure during diastole.

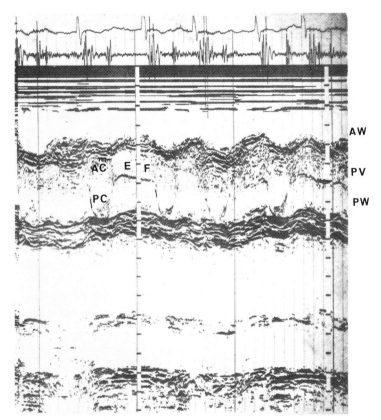

Figure 10–14. Severe pulmonary hypertension. Both the anterior (AC) and posterior (PC) cusps ex-hibit a coarse fluttering. The A wave is absent, and the E-F slope is virtually flat (AW = anterior pul-monary wall; PV = pulmonic valve; PW = posterior pulmonary wall).

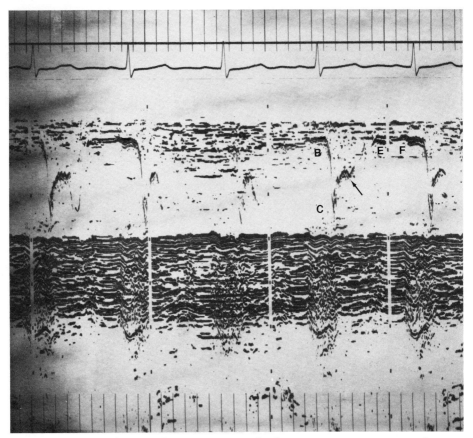

Figure 10–15. Severe pulmonary hypertension. Only the posterior cusp is seen. The A wave is absent, and there is a notch (arrow), with fine fluttering of the leaflet during systole. The E-F slope is markedly flattened, with a significantly increased rate of opening (B-C).

miak et al.,[16] the transducer is placed high, near the left sternal border, and rotated laterally and superiorly from the angle at which the aortic valve is observed. Using the aortic valve as a landmark, the transducer is then angled slightly laterally and superiorly. As the image of the aortic walls disappears, the pulmonary artery becomes visible as an echo-free zone anterior to the aorta (see Figure 10–12). The posterior margin of the pulmonary artery is usually seen as a wide band of echoes 2 to 4 cm behind the anterior margin of the artery. The cusps of the pulmonic valve then appear as thin lines that move between the margins of the pulmonary artery. The space posterior to the pulmonary artery is the lateral aspect of the left atrium.

In a second approach, offered by Weyman et al.,[13] identification of the pulmonic valve is achieved by using the mitral valve as a landmark. By tilting the transducer su-

periorly and slightly toward the throat, the ultrasound beam will pass through the right ventricular outflow tract and the space between the pulmonary artery and the left atrium. With continued upward angulation, the echo-free pulmonary artery will appear 1.0 to 2.0 cm below the anterior wall of the chest. Minute angulations within the pulmonary artery will reveal the valve leaflets.

With either technique, because of the proximity of lung tissue, recording of the pulmonic valve requires that the transducer be tilted in an upward oblique direction. This necessary beam direction explains why the beam usually strikes only the posterior valve cusp. Accurate recordings therefore necessitate that the technologist be very aware of what anatomical structure is being displayed with each particular transducer position. In addition, instrumentation adjustment is particularly critical in view of the fact that the pulmonary artery and valve lie so close to the chest wall. The depth and/or expand controls should be adjusted, extending the echo trace to a position that permits clear visualization of the individual anterior structures. The near gain should then be reduced only to the point at which the heavy anterior echoes are reduced and the finer echoes are delineated.

Associated Pulmonic Abnormalities

Pulmonary Hypertension

When the pressure within the pulmonary artery becomes elevated, the normal configuration of the pulmonary valve is altered. A characteristic feature of the pulmonic valve in patients with severe pulmonary hypertension is a reduced E-F slope. As opposed to the normal "oblique" motion, the diastolic motion (E-F slope) in pulmonary hypertension exhibits a flattened appearance (Fig. 10–14).[16] Other observed features include a decreased or absent A wave, abnormal mid-systolic fluttering and notching, and a significant increase in the opening (B-C) slope (Fig. 10–15).[14]

REFERENCES

1. Hurst JW, and Logue RE (eds.): *The Heart*. New York, McGraw-Hill Book Company, 1970.
2. Joyner CR, Hey EB, and Johnson J: Reflected ultrasound in the diagnosis of tricuspid stenosis. Am J Cardiol 19:66, 1967.
3. Friedewald VE Jr.: *Textbook of Echocardiography*. Philadelphia, W.B. Saunders Company, 1977.
4. Lundström N-R: Echocardiography in the diagnosis of Ebstein's anomaly of the tricuspid valve. Circulation 47:597–605, 1973.
5. Nanda NC, Gramiak R, Shah PM, and Robinson T: Echocardiographic diagnosis of pulmonary hypertension. Excerpt Med 277:12, 1973.
6. Nanda NC, Gramiak R, and Manning JA: Echocardiographic studies of the tricuspid valve in atrial septal defect. *In* White D (Ed.): *Ultrasound in Medicine*. New York, Plenum Press, 1975, pp. 11–17.
7. Waider W, Madry R, McLaurin L, and Craige E: Genesis of right sided heart sounds (Abstr). Circulation (Suppl IV) 7,8:63, 1973.
8. Nanda NC, Gramiak R, and Manning JA: Echocardiography of the tricuspid valve in congenital left ventricular–right atrial communication. Circulation 51:268–272, 1975.
9. Chandraratna PAN, Lopez JM, Fernandez JJ, and Cohen LS: Echocardiographic detection of tricuspid valve prolapse. Circulation 51:823–826, 1975.
10. Tajik AJ, Gau GT, Giuliani ER, Ritter EG, and Schattenberg TT: Echocardiogram in Ebstein's anomaly with Wolff-Parkinson-White preexcitation syndrome, Type B, Circulation 47:813–815, 1973.
11. Kotler MN: Tricuspid valve in Ebstein's anomaly (Letter to the Editor). Circulation 49:194, 1974.
12. Lundström N-R: Ultrasoundcardiography in the diagnosis of Ebstein's anomaly of the tricuspid valve: Preliminary observations. Proc Assoc Europ Pediatr Cardiol 7:44, 1971.
13. Weyman AE, Dillon JC, Feigenbaum H, and Chang S: Echocardiographic patterns of pulmonic valve motion in pulmonary valvular stenosis. Am J Cardiol 34:644–651, 1974.
14. Weyman AE, Dillon JC, Feigenbaum H, and Chang S: Echocardiographic patterns of pulmonic valve motion with pulmonary hypertension. Circulation 50:905–910, 1974.
15. Nanda NC, Gramiak R, Robinson TL, and Shah PM: Echocardiographic evaluation of pulmonary hypertension. Circulation 50:575–581, 1974.
16. Gramiak R, Nanda NC, and Shah PM: Echocardiographic detection of the pulmonary valve. Radiology 102:153–157, 1972.

Chapter 11

PERICARDIAL FLUID

Because the interface between the lung and pericardium produces the dominant echo in the region of the posterior left ventricular wall,[1, 2] it is easily identifiable on the echocardiogram. When fluid accumulates in the pericardial sac, an additional space is created between visceral and parietal pericardium. The detection of the presence of this excess fluid in the pericardial sac is one of the most important applications of echocardiography.

THE PERICARDIUM

The pericardium is a loose-fitting sac of tough, white fibrous tissue that encloses the heart. It is lined with a double layer of serous membrane, consisting of the parietal pericardium and the visceral pericardium, which is adjacent to the outer layer of the heart itself, the epicardium. Between these two membranes is 30 to 50 cc of clear fluid, which lubricates the membrane surfaces and prevents friction between them as the heart contracts.[3]

The actual wall of the heart, the myocardium, which is composed of cardiac muscle, is contiguous with the visceral pericardium. The innermost lining of the myocardium is a thin connective tissue membrane, the endocardium.

A-Mode Appearance

On the A-mode, the posterior wall of the heart in the normal adult appears on the oscilloscope as the most posterior moving cluster of spikes. In the presence of a pericardial effusion, however, the close grouping of these signals is broken by an

echo-free space. On such a recording, the anterior group of signals represents the posterior wall and the visceral pericardium. These signals appear weaker and lower in amplitude than the visceral pericardium–lung interface echoes, which are posterior to the echo-free space (Fig. 11–1).

The anterior wall of the heart in the normal subject is represented by a relatively close grouping of signals that are approximately equal in amplitude and often merging with the "main bang" echoes of the chest wall. These signals arise from the anterior pericardium and the wall of the right ventricle. In the presence of a pericardial effusion, the anterior wall echoes are often distinctly separated from the chest wall by a clear space representing fluid (Fig. 11–2).[4] When such fluid is loculated anteriorly, the anterior echo-free zone may be present, but without evidence of fluid posteriorly. Otherwise, anterior fluid is generally associated with a posterior accumulation.

M-Mode Appearance

Although it is possible to visualize a pericardial effusion on the A-mode, it is most easily recognized on the M-mode, where motion of the ventricular walls can be clearly identified.

In the normal heart, the visceral pericardium and the parietal pericardium are so closely adherent that they appear as a single echo. When fluid accumulates in the pericardial space, however, these surfaces diverge, and abnormal interfaces are created.

Viewed on the M-mode, the echoes from both the relatively static parietal pericardium and the moving visceral pericardium are evident. Between these echoes is an

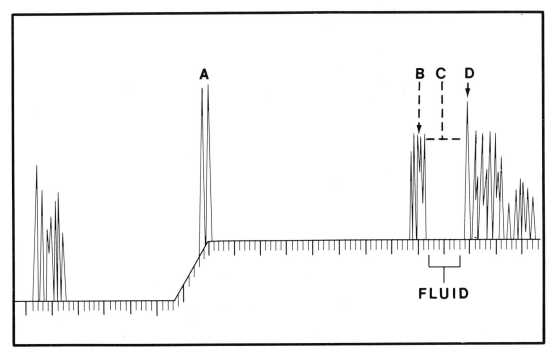

Figure 11–1. A-mode appearance of posterior pericardial fluid. The echoes designated A originate from the interventricular septum. B is a small group of echoes originating from the posterior haert wall and the epicardium. C, an echo-free space, is indicative of the fluid, and D is a cluster of echoes from the pericardium and lung.

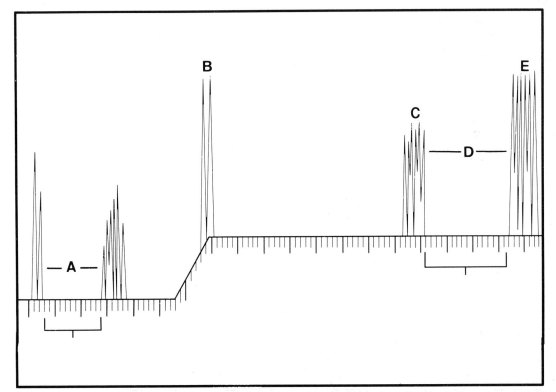

Figure 11–2. A-mode representation of anterior and posterior pericardial fluid. Seen between the anterior heart wall and the wall of the right ventricle, the echo-free space designated A represents the presence of fluid. B originates from the interventricular septum. C originates from the posterior heart wall and the epicardium. D, an echo-free space, represents the fluid, and E is a cluster of echoes originating from the pericardium and lung.

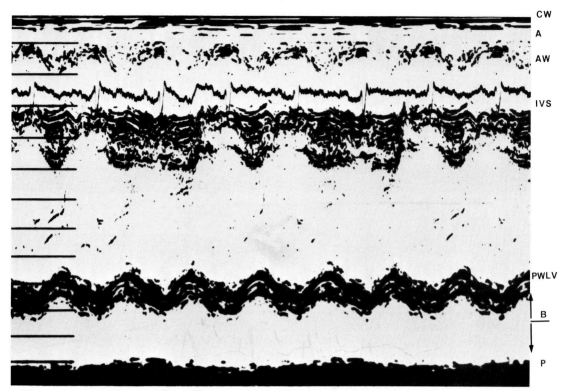

CW
A
AW
IVS
PWLV
B
P

Figure 11–3. Anterior and posterior pericardial fluid. A designates an echo-free space representative of fluid between the anterior heart wall (AW) and the anterior chest wall (CW). B designates an echo-free space representative of fluid between the posterior left ventricular wall (PWLV) and the lung-pericardium interface (P). Note the lack of motion in the pericardium (IVS = interventricular septum).

echo-free space indicative of pericardial fluid. In general, the width of the echo-free space correlates with the amount of fluid present, but precise quantification may not be reliably achieved.[5] When the effusion is very extensive, there is an additional echo-free space between the anterior heart wall echo and the anterior chest wall echo (Fig. 11–3).[4, 6] Except in rare instances in which loculated fluid is detected only anteriorly, the absence of posterior fluid usually excludes the diagnosis of pericardial effusion.

Swinging Heart Motion

In the presence of large collections of fluid, the range of motion of the heart itself increases because it is no longer anchored by the pericardium and is therefore free to rotate about its attachment to the great vessels (Fig. 11–4). As a result, the heart exhibits a swinging motion in which the entire structure, including the anterior wall and the interventricular septum, moves in parallel, anteriorly during ventricular systole and posteriorly during diastole. The removal of even a small amount of the excess pericardial fluid by pericardiocentesis can dramatically alter this abnormal motion.[7]

RECORDING TECHNIQUE

Unless the patient with suspected pericardial effusion experiences difficulty in breathing, there is no reason to deviate from the standard approach to the echocardiographic examination. With the patient in either the supine or the left lateral position, satisfactory test results generally can be obtained. The choice of final placement, however, is often made on the basis of trial and error. Determination of the position of the vertical or horizontal cardiac axis, for example, may lead to changes in transducer placement. (See Chapter 2.)

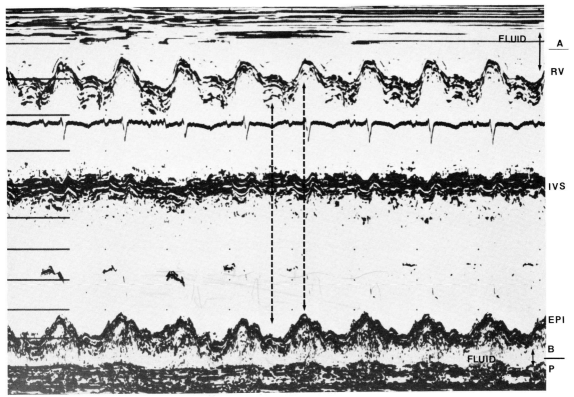

Figure 11–4. Swinging cardiac motion in the presence of a large pericardial effusion. Because of a large accumulation of fluid (A, B), the right ventricular (RV) and left ventricular (LV) echoes demonstrate parallel motion (arrows). This parallel motion of the cardiac walls is characteristic of a large effusion (IVS = interventricular septum; EPI = epicardium; P = pericardium).

The mitral valve serves as an excellent landmark in the identification of the posterior left ventricular wall. Directing the transducer slightly posteriorly, laterally, and inferiorly from the mitral valve will reveal motion that diminishes progressively as the ultrasound beam traverses the left ventricular chamber and encounters the posterior left ventricular wall, which is recognizable by its characteristic motion, anterior in direction during systole and posterior during diastole.

In the presence of a large effusion, the motion of the dominant posterior echo will not parallel the cardiac motion (Fig. 11–3). Instead, there will appear a second, more anterior echo of lower intensity that will show anterior motion with ventricular contraction. The two echoes are separated by the pericardial fluid.

Similarly, an echo-free space may appear between the anterior chest wall and the an-terior wall of the myocardium. Usually fluid in this area is more difficult to detect than posterior fluid, because with the patient in the supine position, the dependent area is posterior to the heart.

The Sector Scan

Further substantiation of pericardial fluid is facilitated by use of the sector scan or "sweep." This recording technique involves identification of the aortic root in the usual manner. Then as the transducer is tilted slightly laterally, inferiorly, and posteriorly, the ultrasound beam will traverse the left atrial chamber, the mitral orifice, and the left ventricular chamber and ultimately will strike the posterior left ventricular wall. The echo-free space indicative of pericardial fluid will become apparent as the beam traverses the atrioventricular

Text continued on page 233

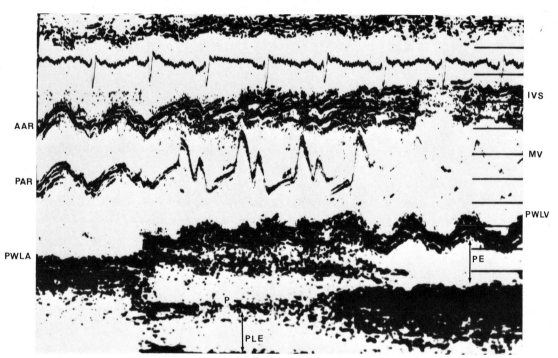

Figure 11–5. Sector scan from the aortic root, to the mitral valve (MV), to the left ventricle. The scan from the aortic root down to the mitral valve reveals an echo-free space where the ultrasonic beam traverses the atrioventricular groove. (As the beam is directed further into the left ventricle, simultaneous pericardial (PE) and pleural (PLE) effusions are separated by an echo (P) from the parietal pericardium and parietal pleura (see Figure 11–6) (AAR = anterior aortic root wall; PAR = posterior aortic root wall; PWLA = posterior wall of the left atrium; PWLV = posterior wall of the left ventricle; IVS = interventricular septum; L = lung).

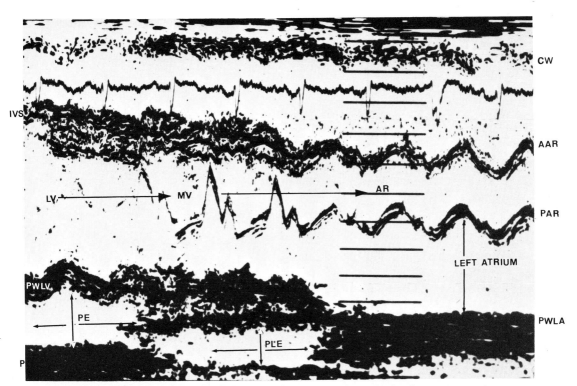

Figure 11–6. Sector scan from the left ventricle (LV), to the mitral valve (MV), to the aortic root. Evidence of the posterior pericardial effusion (PE) diminishes as the ultrasound beam leaves the area of the left ventricle and the atrioventricular groove and disappears completely as the beam traverses the aortic root (AR) and the left atrium. The echo-free space (PLE), indicative of a pleural effusion, also diminishes considerably as the ultrasound beam traverses the left atrium (IVS = interventricular septum; PWLV = posterior wall of the left ventricle; P = pericardium; CW = chest wall; AAR = anterior aortic root wall; PAR = posterior aortic root wall; PWLA = posterior wall of the left atrium).

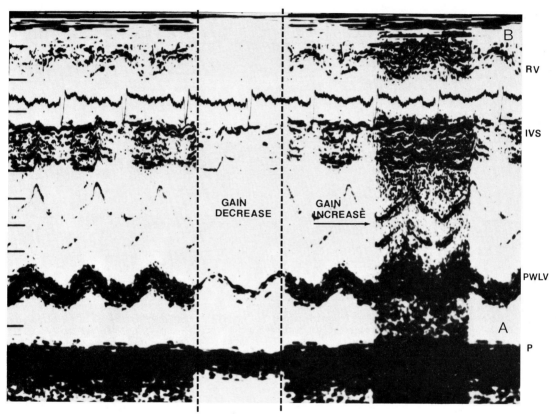

Figure 11–7.   The effect of gain on the appearance of pericardial fluid. In addition to the pronounced posterior echo-free space (A), there is an anterior echo-free zone (B) indicative of a pericardial effusion. As the gain is increased, the echo-free space appears to fill in (arrow). Sonolucent areas do, however, continue to be apparent (RV = right ventricle; IVS = interventricular septum; PWLV = posterior wall of the left ventricle; P = pericardium).

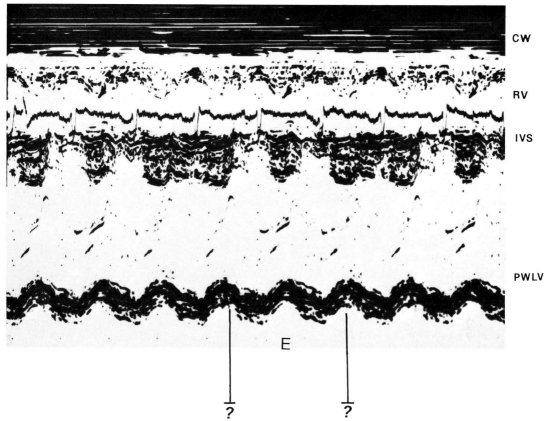

Figure 11–8. With excessive use of the expand (depth) control, the pericardial echoes are not recorded because the display exceeds the range of the oscilloscope. In this view, the severity of the effusion (E) cannot be assessed with accuracy and could be missed entirely (see Figure 11–9) (CW = chest wall; RV = right ventricle; IVS = interventricular septum; PWLV = posterior wall of the left ventricle).

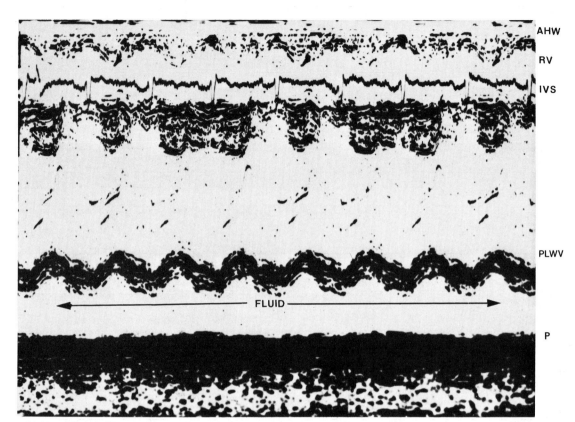

Figure 11–9. Correct use of the expand control. In this view, the posterior echoes are clearly identified (AHW = anterior heart wall; RV = right ventricle; IVS = interventricular septum; PWLV = posterior wall of the left ventricle; P = pericardium).

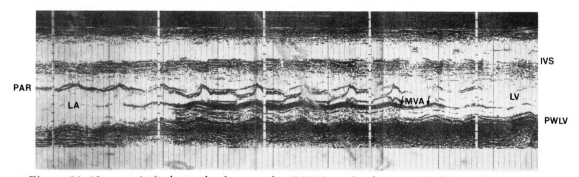

Figure 11–10. A calcified mitral valve annulus (MVA) can be distinguished from the posterior left ventricular wall (PWLV) when sweeping from the left atrium (LA) to the left ventricle (LV), thus eliminating the possibility of pseudo pericardial fluid (PAR = posterior aortic root; IVS = interventricular septum).

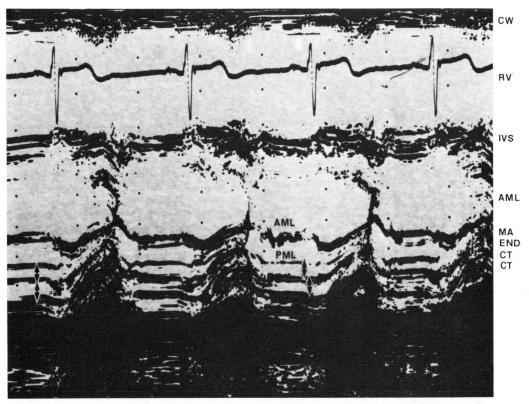

Figure 11-11.   Directing the transducer too far medially and inferiorly toward the mitral apparatus causes the posterior mitral leaflet (PML), the annulus (MA), the chordae tendineae (CT), and the endocardium (END) to appear as exaggerated, separate structures (arrows). This combination of echoes closely resembles the characteristic findings of a pericardial effusion (CW = chest wall; RV = right ventricle; IVS = interventricular septum; AML = anterior mitral leaflet).

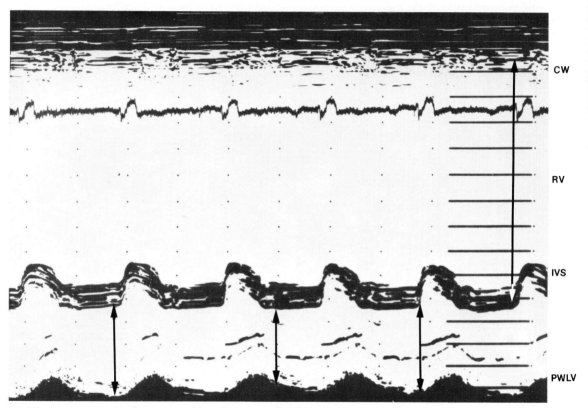

CW

RV

IVS

PWLV

Figure 11–12. Right ventricular volume overload. In the presence of a severely enlarged right ventricle (RV), the septum (IVS) is dramatically displaced and exhibits a motion similar to that of the posterior left ventricular wall (PWLV). The echo-free space (arrows) between the septum and the posterior left ventricular wall could be mistaken for pericardial fluid (CW = chest wall).

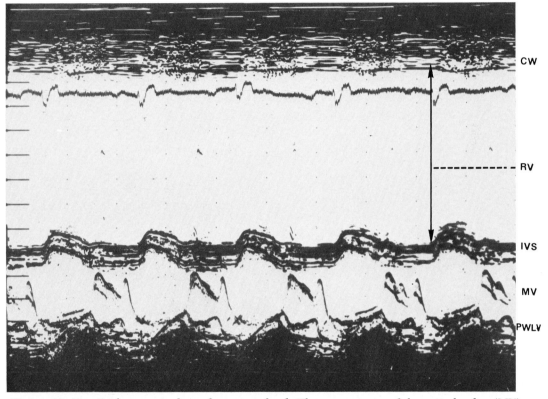

Figure 11–13.   Right ventricular volume overload. The appearance of the mitral valve (MV) posterior to the septum (IVS) obviates the possibility that the posterior left ventricular wall (PWLV) will be mistaken for pericardial fluid (CW = chest wall; RV = right ventricle).

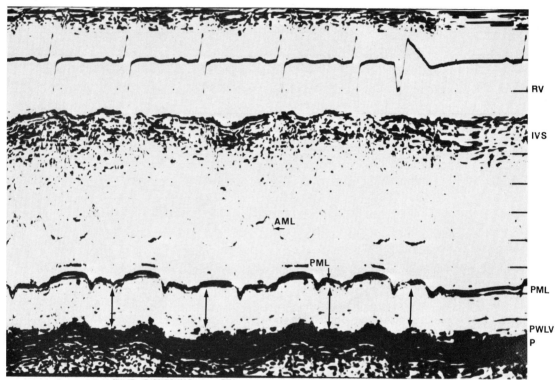

Figure 11–14. Because of abnormal thickening of the posterior mitral valve leaflet (PML), it appears as a heavy echo running immediately anterior to the posterior left ventricular wall (PWLV). The anterior mitral leaflet (AML) is barely visible. The echo-free space (arrows) between the posterior mitral leaflet and the posterior left ventricular wall (PWLV) must not be mistaken for a pericardial effusion. Note the good contractility of the posterior left ventricular wall and the pericardium (P) (RV = right ventricle; IVS = interventricular septum).

groove (Fig. 11–5). On the sweep back from the posterior left ventricular wall and up to the aortic root, the echo-free area will gradually disappear as the ultrasound beam again intersects the left atrial wall (Fig. 11–6).

When the ultrasound beam is focused on the posterior wall of the left ventricle, gain studies should be performed. This is accomplished by reducing the gain until the posterior wall appears as a single echo. The gain should then gradually be increased until the myocardial-pericardial echoes are visualized. If an echo-free space remains between the epicardial and pericardial surfaces, this must be considered strong evidence of a fluid-filled area (Fig. 11–7).

PULMONARY DISEASE

In subjects with pulmonary emphysema, posterior pericardial fluid is sometimes difficult to detect, and the dominant posterior wall signal may not be identified clearly. The hyperaerated lung interposed between the chest wall and the heart interferes with direct recording of the cardiac echoes. In such cases, an adequate scan may be obtained only if a recording is made from the subxyphoid position. (See Chapter 2.)

Large pleural effusions produce a space usually in excess of 4 cm between the echoes of the posterior heart and the air-filled lung.[1] It is not unusual to see both a pleural effusion and a pericardial effusion in the acutely ill patient. For this reason, when pericardial fluid is identified, it is good practice to examine the area posterior to this fluid for signs of a second echo-free space indicative of pleural fluid (Figs. 11–6 and 11–7).

CAUSES OF PERICARDIAL FLUID ABNORMALITIES

Pericardial effusions may develop slowly in association with chronic renal disease, liver failure, tumor irradiation, or infections of the pericardium. Sudden accumulation of fluid in the pericardium may occur following thoracic surgery or chest injury. When an effusion is acute, cardiac function may be impaired by the direct compression of the heart; this is termed cardiac tamponade. Whatever the cause of an effusion, the chest x-ray may demonstrate only an enlarging cardiac silhouette, whereas the echocardiogram allows for differentiation of enlargement from pericardial fluid accumulation.

Examples of various technical errors demonstrating pseudo pericardial effusions are shown in Figures 11–8 to 11–14.

REFERENCES

1. Goldberg BB, Ostrum BJ, and Isaac HJ: Ultrasonic determination of pericardial effusion. JAMA 202:927–930, 1967.
2. Soulen RL. Lapayowker MS, and Cortes FM: Distribution of pericardial fluid: Dynamic and static influences. Am J Roentgenol Rad Ther Nucl Med 103:583–588, 1969.
3. Klein JJ, Raber G, Shimada H, Kingsley B, and Segal BL: Evaluation of induced pericardial effusion by reflected ultrasound. Am J Cardiol 22:49. 1968.
4. Edler I: Diagnostic use of ultrasound in heart disease. Acta Med Scand 308:32–36, 1955.
5. Gramiak R, and Shah PM: Cardiac ultrasonography. Radiol Clin North Am 9:469, 1971.
6. Feigenbaum H, Zaky A, and Waldhausen JA: Use of ultrasound in the diagnosis of pericardial effusion. Ann Intern Med 65:443–452, 1966.
7. Littmann D, and Spodick DH: Total electrical alternation in pericardial disease. Circulation 13:912, 1958.

Chapter 12

PROSTHETIC VALVES

Physicians have been faced with the problem of assessing the functional integrity and performance of prosthetic valves since their first placement in the human heart. Among the techniques employed in this evaluation, echocardiography is probably potentially the best single means for obtaining accurate studies. There are, however, limitations to current ultrasound techniques that must be clearly defined.

A major problem confronting the investigator is the wide structural variance among the models of prosthetic valves available. Obviously, each different valve type has its own unique echocardiographic features. Furthermore, identical valves placed in different anatomical positions will have different echocardiographic appearances, because the transducer beam strikes the valves from different angles and contacts different interfaces of the structures. To evaluate the function of the valve accurately, its component parts must be identified on the echocardiogram. It is therefore imperative that the physician and the technologist be familiar with the basic design of each type of prosthesis.

As an aid to better understanding of the echocardiographic analysis of prosthetic valve motion, studies referred to as "in-vitro," which means outside of the body, have been conducted to artificially simulate valvular prostheses. These in-vitro studies of the echocardiographic M-mode features of various types of prostheses have been reported from several different sources.[1, 2] The model for such investigations consists of a saline-filled chamber in which a prosthetic valve is mounted. The ball or disc of the valve is activated by the flow of saline solution across the valve. Recordings of the

valve are taken from angles of zero to 90 degrees to the suture ring of the valve and from several points around the circumference of the valve ring (Fig. 12–1).

In the studies reported by Ellis et al.[1] and Johnson et al.,[2] the various component parts of the valves were easily identified and correlated with in-vivo (in the living body) echocardiographic recordings. The beam angle of the transducer in all cases was shown to be of critical importance. Maximum disc or ball excursion was obtained at or near an angle of 90 degrees, where the disc or poppet moved directly toward and away from the transducer beam. This transducer angle approximates the positions employed in visualizing prosthetic valves in the mitral position. As the angle approaches zero degrees, the disc or poppet moves in and out of the transducer beam with little or no trackable motion of the moving component. This angle most closely simulates the in-vivo recording of the prosthetic valve in the aortic position.

Evaluation includes both immediate and long-term follow-up recordings of the mechanical function of the prosthesis in all patients. Comparison of initial postoperative recordings with later studies will reveal changes in the excursion of the disc or poppet as well as alterations in wall motion and in the size of any of the cardiac chambers, any of which could be indicative of a malfunctioning valve.

It is important to note that some degree of regurgitation occurs in all artificial heart valves during the closing delay. In a study by Bjork et al.,[3] the total amount of regurgitation was lowest with the Starr-Edwards valve at 3 per cent. The Kay-Shiley valve showed regurgitation at 4 per cent; the

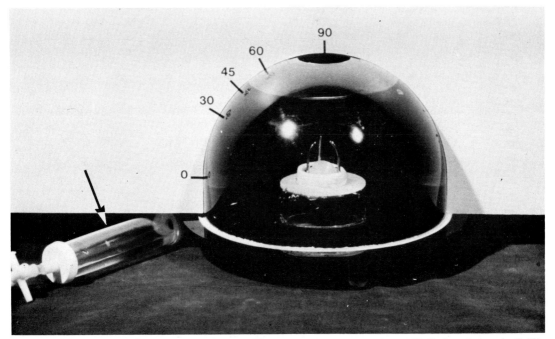

Figure 12–1. A Smeloff-Cutter valve prosthesis mounted in a saline-filled chamber. The ball is activated by the hand pump (arrow), which produces flow of the saline solution across the valve. *In vitro* studies are performed by placing the transducer on the face of the chamber using a coupling gel and directing it toward the prosthesis from various angles. (Courtesy of Human Prosthetics, Cutter Laboratories, Inc.)

Smeloff-Cutter at 7 per cent; the Bjork-Shiley at 10 per cent; and the Wada-Cutter at 25 per cent.

RECORDING THE PROSTHETIC VALVE

There is no standardized chest wall position from which all prosthetic valves can be satisfactorily recorded. As a general rule, the optimal position is the one from which the maximum excursion of the disc or poppet can be recorded. Transducer angulation is particularly critical because variations affect the overall valve appearance as well as the amplitude of excursion of the moving component. Therefore, recordings must be taken from several angles to ensure that the maximum excursion is recorded.

On the A-mode, several distinct echoes can be visualized. One must identify both those echoes from the fixed structures whose movement is caused solely by the motion of the entire heart and those originating from the disc or poppet, which has its own independent motion.

Echoes reflected from the prosthetic valve components are usually quite strong and are sometimes difficult to delineate.

Therefore, it is necessary to attentuate the echoes by increasing either the amount of reject control or overall gain in order to clarify the echoes that originate from the entire valve structure. A recording should be made only when individual echoes from the different components of the prosthesis appear on the A-mode display. (The specific characteristic patterns of each type of prosthesis are described in the sections titled "Echocardiographic Appearance" throughout this chapter.)

THE ELECTROCARDIOGRAM AND THE PROSTHETIC VALVE

A simultaneous electrocardiogram is extremely important in the identification and timing of the independently moving echoes of a prosthetic valve. Its opening and closing should occur at approximately the same point in the cardiac cycle as the normal cardiac valve. Delayed opening of the valve could be indicative of clot or pannus formation; early opening could be the result of a paraprosthetic leak.

Correlation of the electrocardiogram can establish whether the independently moving echoes of the prosthetic valve show mo-

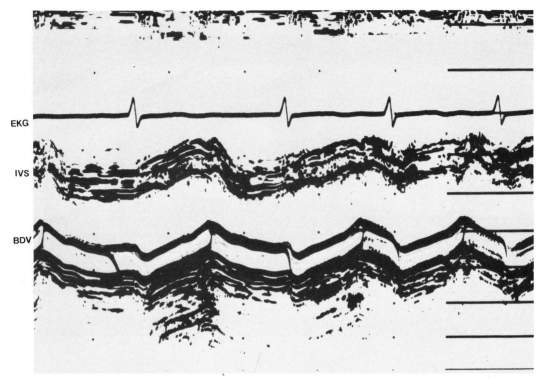

Figure 12–2.   M-mode tracing of a Beall mitral prosthesis demonstrating the rhythm disturbance of a patient in atrial fibrillation. Note the differences in the duration of opening of each beat (EKG = electrocardiogram; IVS = interventricular septum; BDV = Beall disc valve).

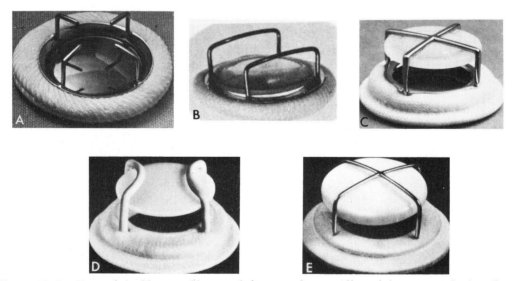

Figure 12–3.   Examples of low-profile mitral disc prostheses. All models consist of a free-floating disc, cage struts, and a suture ring. (A) Cooley-Cutter. (B) Beall Model 106. (C) Starr-Edwards. (D) Beall Model 103. (E) Harken. (A — Courtesy of Human Prosthetics, Cutter Laboratories, Inc.; B, D, E — Courtesy of Surgitool, Travenol Laboratories, Inc., Artificial Organs Division; C — Courtesy of Edwards Laboratories, Division of American Hospital Supply.)

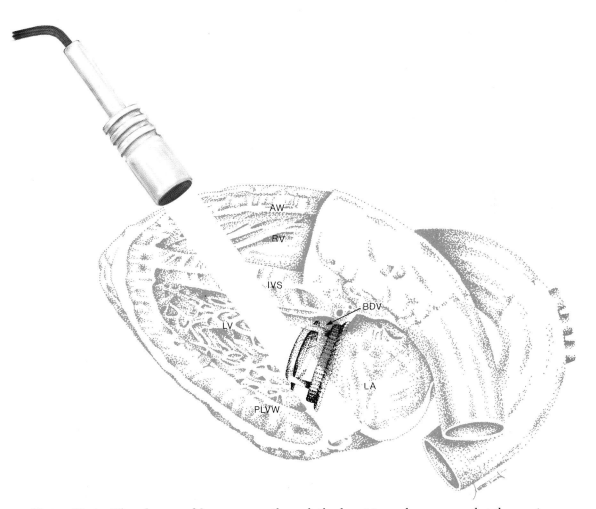

Figure 12–4. The ultrasound beam passes through the heart in such a manner that the maximum excursion of the disc is recorded. A Beall disc valve is shown in this illustration (AW = anterior heart wall; RV = right ventricle; IVS = interventricular septum; LV = left ventricle; PWLV = posterior left ventricular wall; BDV = Beall disc valve; LA = left atrium). (Beall disc valve courtesy of Surgitool, Travenol Laboratories, Inc., Artificial Organs Division.)

tion toward or away from the transducer in each phase of the cardiac cycle. This determination is an invaluable aid in establishing the angle at which the transducer beam is striking the prosthesis. Just as arrhythmias affect the normal mitral and aortic valves (see Chapter 3), they also affect the motion of the prosthetic valve. For example, Alderman et al.,[4] describe a "fluttering" of the mitral poppet in mid- to late diastole in a patient in atrial flutter. Many patients undergoing valve replacement are in atrial fibrillation in which the rhythm is grossly irregular (Fig. 12–2). Therefore, at least 10 consecutive heartbeats should be recorded to demonstrate repeated opening and closing motions of the prosthetic valve.

THE DISC MITRAL PROSTHETIC VALVE

Valve Design

The disc valve is used principally in the mitral position. The valve consists of a free-floating disc with a Teflon or silicon rubber surface, cage struts, and usually a Dacron-covered base and suture ring. The principle of the low-profile disc design is to minimize cage protrusion into the left ventricle and to minimize obstruction of the left ventricular outflow tract (Fig. 12–3).

Anatomical Position

The prosthesis is sutured into the mitral annulus with the struts extending into the left ventricle. The disc opens into the left ventricle and moves toward the transducer in ventricular diastole and away from the transducer in systole (Fig. 12–4).

Echocardiographic Appearance

A-Mode

On the A-mode, the disc valve appears as three distinct echoes: (1) the struts, (2) the base and suture ring, and (3) the disc, which moves rapidly between these two echoes with an excursion of from 5 to 7 mm. The thick echoes representing the struts and suture ring move in parallel approximately 1.5 cm apart (Fig. 12–5).

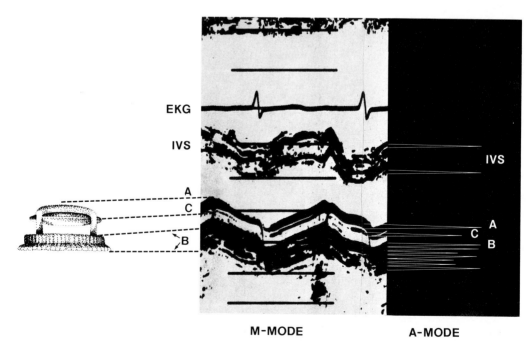

Figure 12–5. M-mode and A-mode representations of the various component parts of the low-profile disc valve. The disc moves anteriorly during diastole and posteriorly with the QRS complex (A = strut; B = base and suture ring; C = disc; IVS = interventricular septum; EKG = electrocardiogram).

M-Mode

On the M-mode, the echoes representing the prosthetic valve are located just posterior to the interventricular septum. The strut echoes and the base and suture ring echoes move in parallel, gradually anteriorly until the end of the electrocardiographic T wave and then posteriorly until the QRS complex. The echo reflected from the disc shows opening motion at the end of the T wave, with a rapid anterior motion converging with the strut echoes. A the time of the QRS complex, the disc closes rapidly with a posterior movement (Fig. 12–5).

Recording Technique

Mitral Disc Prosthesis

Because the mitral valve is a relatively easy structure to record, recording the maximum excursion of the disc of the prosthetic valve in this position is not especially difficult, particularly since its orientation in the heart allows the ultrasound beam to strike the disc parallel to the axis of its motion (see Figure 12–4). Usually, this can be accomplished by positioning the transducer in the normal mitral valve position in the fourth or fifth intercostal space and angling superiorly from the left sternal border.

Care must be taken to record all areas of the valve. Thrombus may form on only one strut, which would restrict the excursion of only one side of the disc. When maximum disc excursion is obtained, angulation of the transducer should be slightly altered, so that the other strut can be visualized. Proper transducer angulation is a critical factor in the evaluation of any prosthetic valve. Incorrect transducer placement or angulation could result in minimizing the excursion of the valve or in making the recording difficult, if not impossible, to evaluate (Fig. 12–6).

Measuring the Mitral Disc Prosthesis

Optimally, measurement of the disc excursion should be made from at least two different edges of the disc, although echocardiographic distinction between the edges is usually quite difficult. Because of the variations in valve sizes, measurements of the component parts of the mitral prostheses differ. For example, the disc excursion can vary from approximately 5 mm in a small Beall valve to 8 mm in a large size. In optimal recordings, measurement of the disc excursion is easily made with the prosthesis in the mitral position, mainly because the ultrasound beam is approximately parallel to the disc motion. Increased attentuation control in some instances is necessary in recording the valve to insure that all parts of the valve are clearly distinguishable for measurement (Fig. 12–7).

It is important to observe the distance between the disc and the base of the valve while it is closed in systole. Failure to close completely can be indicative of thrombus formation around the base of the valve. In addition to the measurements of the prosthesis, all other chambers and valves visualized should be routinely recorded and measured. Changes in the size of the chambers can be indicative of some problem with the function of the prosthetic valve.

THE TILTING DISC AORTIC PROSTHETIC VALVE

Valve Design

Although each of the tilting disc valves commercially available differs somewhat in appearance, the basic configuration is similar. The tilting disc valve consists of a suspended disc that opens on some type of axis to an angle of from 60 to 80 degrees. Each type of valve has an inner metal ring surrounded by a Teflon suture ring (Fig. 12–8).

Anatomical Position

When the tilting disc valve is placed in the aortic position, it is sutured into the aortic annulus with the larger edge of the disc opening into the aorta. In some replacements, the larger portion of the disc opens away from the anterior wall of the aortic root (Fig. 12–9). The valve can also be sutured into the aortic annulus with the larger portion of the disc opening away from the posterior, or left atrial side, of the aortic root (Fig. 12–10). The orientation of the disc will not influence the function of the valve as

Text continued on page 245

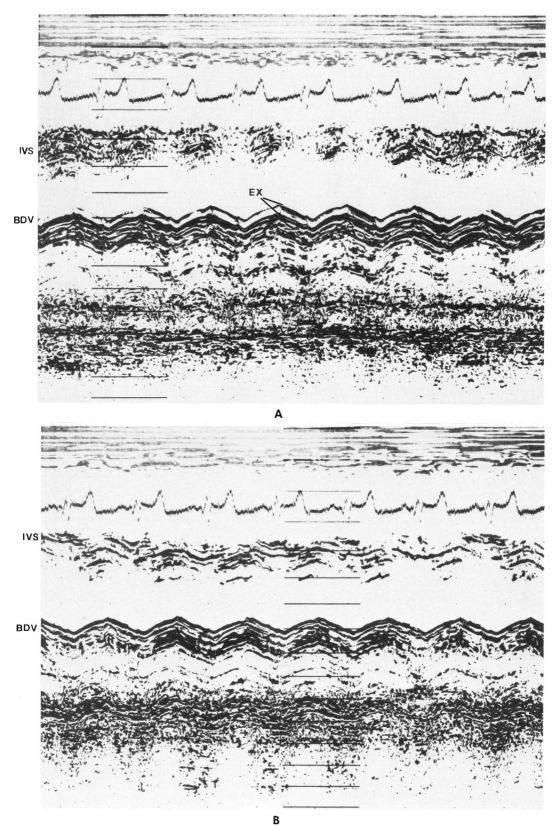

Figure 12-6. (A) M-mode recording illustrating how improper angulation can result in the appearance of a reduction in the excursion (EX) of the valve. (B) M-mode recording illustrating how improper transducer angulation can produce echoes that make distinguishing the individual component parts of the prosthesis impossible (IVS = interventricular septum; BDV = Beall disc valve).

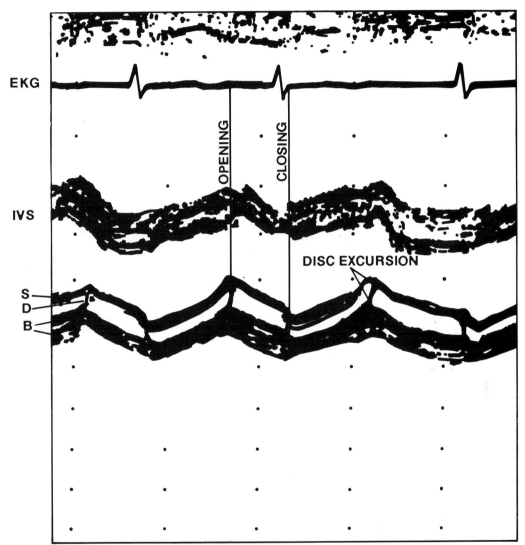

Figure 12-7.   M-mode illustration of a disc mitral prosthesis indicating the points of measurement of the disc excursion and the opening and closing of the disc in reference to the electrocardiogram (EKG) (IVS = interventricular septum; S = strut; D = disc; B = base and suture ring).

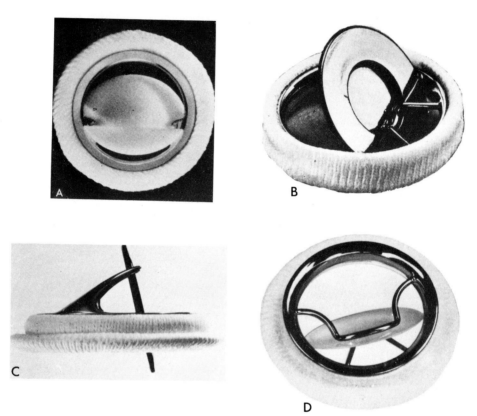

Figure 12–8.   Various commercially available tilting disc prosthetic valves. (A) Wada-Cutter mitral valve prosthesis, 60° opening. (B) Bjork-Shiley aortic valve prosthesis, 60° opening. (C) Lillehei-Kaster mitral valve prosthesis, 80° opening. (D) Bjork-Shiley mitral valve prosthesis, 60° opening. (A–Courtesy of Human Prosthetics, Cutter Laboratories, Inc.; B, D–Courtesy of Shiley Laboratories, Inc.; C–Courtesy of Medical Incorporated.)

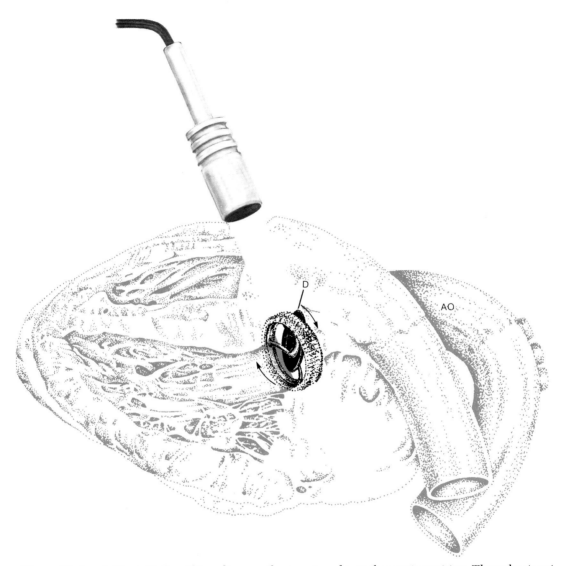

Figure 12–9.   A Bjork-Shiley tilting disc prosthesis sutured into the aortic position. The valve is oriented so that the larger part of the disc (D) opens from the anterior portion of the aortic root into the aorta (AO) and moves toward the posterior aspect of the root as it opens to its full excursion. (Arrows indicate the direction of disc opening.) (Bjork-Shiley tilting disc prosthesis courtesy of Shiley Laboratories, Inc.)

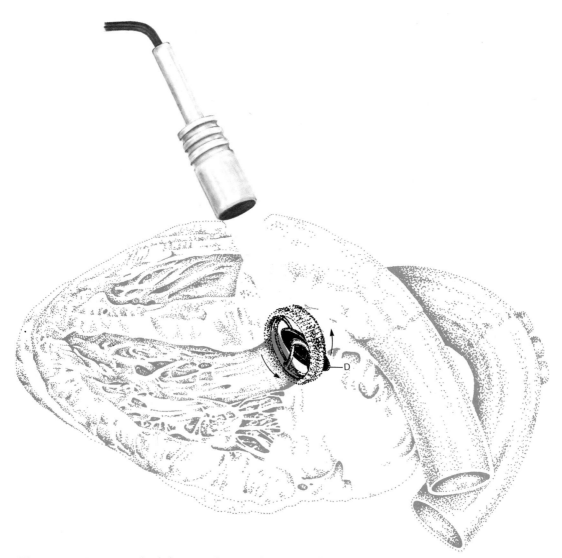

Figure 12–10. A Bjork-Shiley prosthetic valve sutured into the base of the aorta so that the larger portion of the disc (D) opens in a direction from the posterior aortic root to the anterior portion of the root. In most cases, from this view the echo representing the inferior portion of the disc is not visualized. (Arrows indicate the direction of disc opening.) (Bjork-Shiley prosthetic valve courtesy of Shiley Laboratories, Inc.)

long as the disc is able to move freely. The disc opens from 60 to 80 degrees, depending upon the specific valve used, with the superior edge of the disc extending into the aorta and the inferior edge oriented toward the left ventricular outflow tract.

Echocardiographic Appearance

A-Mode

On the A-mode, with the valve sutured into the annulus as illustrated in Figure 12–9, the tilting disc aortic prosthesis reflects two heavy and distinct signals that represent the suture ring attachments to the anterior and posterior walls of the aortic root and two or three other signals from the valve moving within the aortic root (Fig. 12–11).

The signals representing the anterior and posterior aortic root walls are heavier than normal because of the suture ring but are usually within the normal aortic root dimensions of 28 to 40 mm. Moving within the aortic root and suture ring during systole are three distinct signals: (1) the echoes originating from the anterior edge of the disc, (2) those reflecting from the metal struts, and (3) those from the posterior edge of the disc.

With the disc valve sutured into the aortic annulus as illustrated in Figure 12–10, the A-mode appearance is similar to that just described. However, an echo representing the larger portion of the disc is seen moving anteriorly during systole rather than posteriorly.

M-Mode

On the M-mode recordings, with the disc valve oriented in the aortic position facing the anterior aortic root as shown in Figure 12–9, the disc is represented by three or four strong horizontal signals appearing within the aortic root and suture ring during systole (Figs. 12–12 and 12–13). The signals representing the anterior and posterior walls of the aortic root appear heavier than normal because of the presence of the suture ring. The diameter of the suture ring in the tilting disc prosthesis can vary from 17 to 32 mm, and on an optimal recording, it can be distinguished from the aortic root.

Ordinarily, the transducer beam will strike the valve in such a way that as it opens, the larger edge of the disc moves posteriorly and the smaller edge of the disc moves anteriorly. In the closed position during diastole, three main echoes are seen: (1) the anterior aortic root and suture ring, (2) the echo from the metal struts, and (3) the posterior aortic root and suture ring. When oriented in the aortic annulus as shown in Figure 12–10, the tilting disc pros-

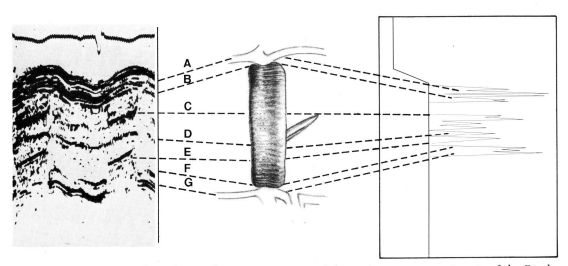

Figure 12–11. M-mode and A-mode representations of the various component parts of the Bjork-Shiley tilting disc valve (A = anterior aortic root; B = anterior suture ring; C = superior edge of disc; D = metal strut; E = inferior edge of disc; F = posterior suture ring; G = posterior aortic root).

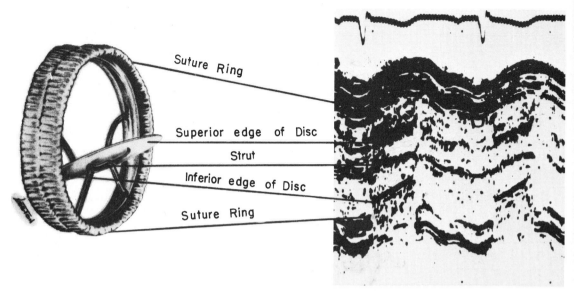

Figure 12–12. Identification of the various component parts of an M-mode tracing of a Bjork-Shiley aortic valve prosthesis.

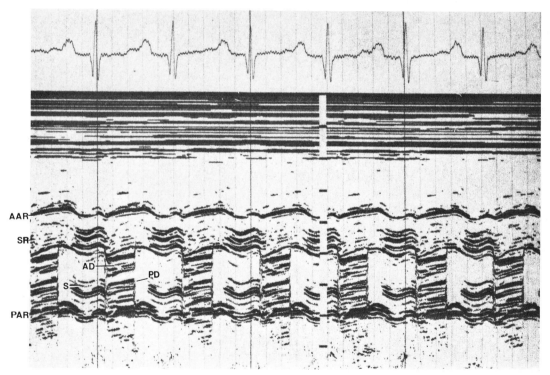

Figure 12–13. M-mode representation of a #14 Lillehei-Kaster prosthetic valve sutured into the aortic annulus in a way similar to the valve orientation shown in Figure 12–9. As the tilting disc moves to its open position, one edge of the disc moves posteriorly, or away from the ultrasound beam, and the other edge of the disc moves anteriorly, or toward the beam (AAR = anterior aortic root; SR = suture ring; AD = anterior disc edge; PD = posterior disc edge; S = metal strut; PAR = posterior aortic root wall).

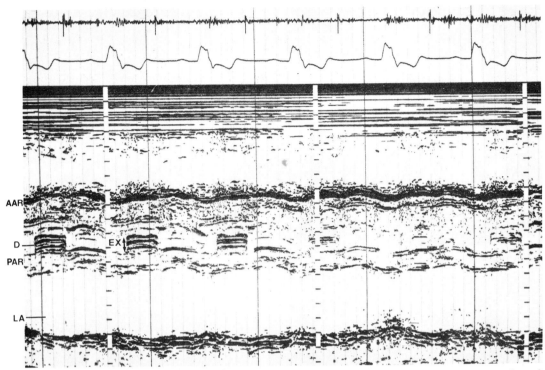

Figure 12–14.   M-mode representation of a #29 Bjork-Shiley tilting disc valve positioned in the aortic annulus with the larger portion of the disc opening into the aorta toward the anterior wall of the aortic root as in Figure 12–10. The excursion of this disc (EX) is approximately 12 mm (AAR = anterior aortic root; D = disc; PAR = posterior aortic root wall; LA = left atrium).

thesis produces a slightly different appearance on the M-mode (Fig. 12–14). Within the aortic root, the larger edge of the disc is seen moving from the posterior aortic root anteriorly. From this view, with the Bjork-Shiley prosthesis, the posterior excursion of the smaller portion of the disc usually is not visualized. The continuous echoes appearing in the center of the aortic root represent the struts of the valve. The apparent excursion of the disc is dependent upon the size of the prosthesis used and the angle from which the valve is recorded. Again, the optimal recording is that in which the greatest excursion of the disc is observed.

In an *in-vitro* (simulated) study by Ellis et al.,[1] a Bjork-Shiley No. 27 aortic prosthesis was mounted in a saline-filled chamber. Ultrasound recordings were taken from angles of zero degrees to 90 degrees relative to the suture ring of the valve and from four different view points around the circumference of the valve ring (Fig. 12–15). These recordings were then compared with *in-vivo* echocardiograms from patients with

the Bjork-Shiley prosthesis in both the mitral and the aortic positions. The results showed that the *in-vitro* (simulated) recordings of this valve that corresponded most directly with the *in-vivo* echocardiograms of patients with this type of aortic valve replacement sutured into the aortic annulus as shown in Figure 12–9 were obtained from position A at an angle of zero to 5 degrees (Fig. 12–16).

In the study, the larger edge of the disc appeared approximately 10 mm from the anterior suture ring, exclusive of the width of the aortic root. One or both of the metal struts lay approximately 10 to 15 mm from the suture ring, depending upon the angulation and the position of the transducer. Position A gave the greatest distance, and position D gave the least. The echo from the struts appeared as a single uninterrupted line moving anteriorly with systole and posteriorly with diastole as the aorta itself moved with the heart. The echo of the smaller portion of the disc appeared approximately 5 to 8 mm from the posterior suture

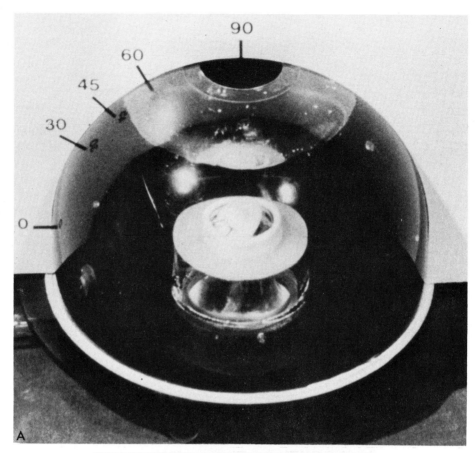

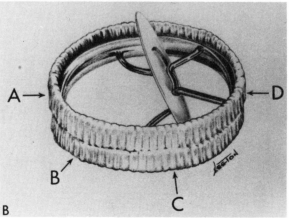

Figure 12–15. (A) A saline-filled chamber with a Bjork-Shiley #27 prosthesis mounted in the center. A hand pump is used to activate flow across the valve, simulating its opening and closing motion. (B) Bjork-Shiley prosthetic valve with the four positions, A, B, C, and D, identified around the circumference of the valve ring. (Courtesy of Shiley Laboratories, Inc.)

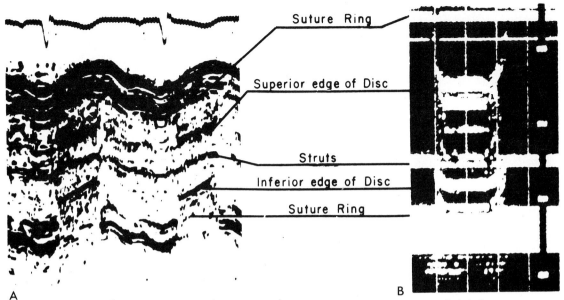

Figure 12–16. (A) The *in vivo* M-mode recording shown in comparison with (B) the *in vitro* recording from the valve chamber.

ring, again excluding the width of the aortic root. It is important to recognize that the position of these echoes will vary with angulation changes and with differences in the size of the prosthesis used.

With the Bjork-Shiley aortic prosthesis sutured into the aortic annulus as shown in Figure 12–10, the *in-vitro* recording obtained from the valve chamber that was most closely related to the *in-vivo* tracing taken from a patient was obtained from an angle of approximately zero degrees to 5 degrees from position D.

Recording Technique

Aortic Prosthesis

Using the anterior mitral valve leaflet as a landmark, the transducer should be angled slightly superiorly and medially until the mitral valve loses its characteristic motion and the two distinctive spikes of the anterior and posterior aortic root walls appear on the A-mode. From this point, slight manipulation of the transducer may be necessary to bring in the motion of the disc as it opens and closes. Also, severe use of the attenuation and reject controls will be necessary to reduce the abnormally heavy echoes originating from the prosthetic valve. These adjustments are critical, and caution should be exercised to not eliminate the echoes from the posterior atrial wall that are necessary for measurement of the left atrium. Several recordings utilizing different transducer angulations and varying attenuation levels should be made to allow for thorough evaluation of the valve prosthesis.

THE TILTING DISC MITRAL PROSTHETIC VALVE

Valve Design

The design of each of the available prostheses varies only slightly when used in the mitral position. The difference lies mainly in the construction of the suture ring and does not significantly alter the echocardiographic appearance of the valve.

Anatomical Position

The valve is sutured into the mitral annulus with the larger portion of the disc opening into the left ventricle and the smaller portion extending into the left atrium (Fig. 12–17). Two positions of orientation of the valve in the mitral annulus

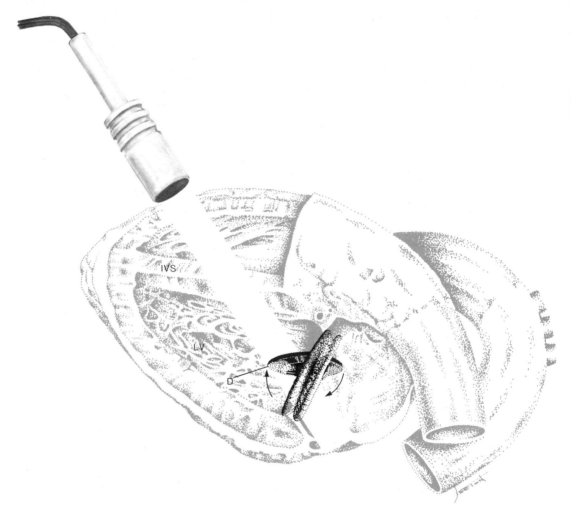

Figure 12–17. An illustration of a Bjork-Shiley mitral valve prosthesis in the mitral position. The valve is sutured into the mitral annulus so that the larger portion of the disc (D) opens into the left ventricle (LV) and toward the interventricular septum (IVS). (Arrows indicate the direction of disc opening.) (Bjork-Shiley mitral valve prosthesis courtesy of Shiley Laboratories, Inc.)

have been described. The earlier method, described by Bjork et al.,[5] was to orient the larger portion of the disc anteriorly, so that the main flow of the valve was toward the ventricular septum. In an article by Reid,[6] it was argued that less energy would be dissipated and the flow pattern would be smoother with the valve oriented so that the flow would be directed toward the posterior wall of the left ventricle as shown in Figure 12–17.

Echocardiographic Appearance

A-Mode

As with any cardiac structure, the appearance of the tilting disc mitral prosthesis on the A-mode varies considerably with transducer angulation. Utilizing the same transducer angulation as in Figure 12–17, the signals from the valve will appear approximately 10 mm posterior to the echoes from the interventricular septum during diastole (Fig. 12–18). The most anterior valve signal will be that of the disc in its fully opened position. This signal will move anteriorly and posteriorly, with an excursion of approximately 7 to 10 mm. Posterior to the disc signal are the heavy echoes originating from the metal struts and the suture ring. These echoes will exhibit an anterior-posterior motion with an excursion of approximately 10 mm with each cardiac cycle. Posterior to the valve echoes are the signals arising from the left ventricular wall. With slight superior angulation of the transducer, the left atrial wall will be seen posterior to the valve signals in place of the left ventricular wall.

M-Mode

On the M-mode, the overall appearance of the tilting disc prosthesis is very similar to that of a stenotic mitral valve (see Figure 12–18). It will be seen moving anteriorly at the end of the electrocardiographic T wave and posteriorly at the end of the QRS complex, with an excursion of approximately 10 mm. The heavy echoes posterior to those of the disc are created by the suture ring and the metal struts. These echoes show only the movement of the heart itself and no independent movement of the structures themselves.

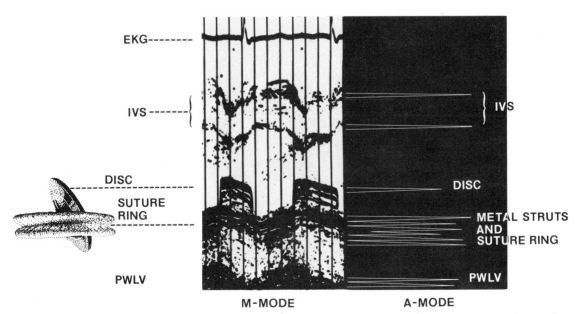

Figure 12–18. M-mode and A-mode representations of the various component parts of the Bjork-Shiley mitral valve prosthesis (IVS = interventricular septum; PWLV = posterior wall of the left ventricle).

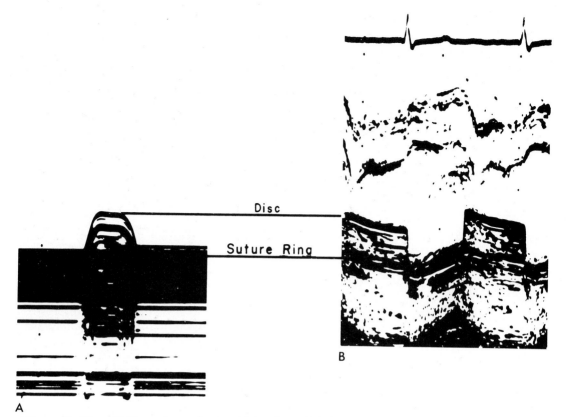

Figure 12–19. (A) The echoes obtained from the valve chamber (*in vitro*) recorded with the transducer in a position of about 80 degrees to the base of the valve (see Figure 12–15) shown in correlation with (B), an M-mode recording of a Bjork-Shiley valve in the mitral position.

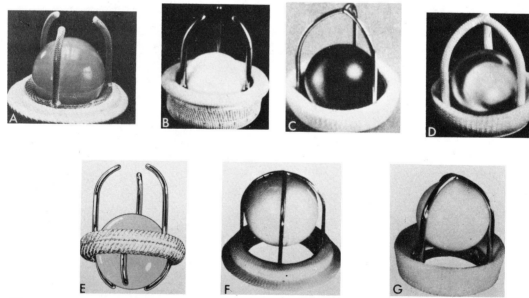

Figure 12–20. Examples of various ball-type prosthetic valves. (A) Braunwald-Cutter mitral valve prosthesis. (B) Magovern-Cromie aortic valve prosthesis. (C) DeBakey Surgitool aortic valve prosthesis. (D) Surgitool aortic valve prosthesis. (E) Smeloff-Cutter aortic valve prosthesis. (F) Starr-Edwards mitral valve prosthesis, Model 6120. (G) Starr-Edwards aortic valve prosthesis, Model 1200. (A, E—Courtesy of Human Prosthesis, Cutter Laboratories, Inc.; B–D—Courtesy of Surgitool, Travenol Laboratories, Inc., Artificial Organs Division; F, G—Courtesy of Edwards Laboratories, Division of American Hospital Supply.)

In the *in-vitro* studies conducted with the saline-filled chamber, as illustrated in Figure 12–15, the ultrasound recording found to relate most directly with the *in-vivo* echocardiogram of a patient with a Bjork-Shiley mitral valve was taken from an angle of approximately 75 degrees to 90 degrees from position D (Fig. 12–19). The excursion of the disc at this transducer position measured 10 mm. The inferior portion of the disc was not observed from this view.

Recording Technique

Mitral Prosthesis

By initially using the A-mode to locate the echoes of the mitral prosthesis, the angulation of the transducer can then be minutely altered to determine the optimal transducer angle. When the individual echoes of the valve can be seen clearly on the A-mode, the attenuation and reject controls should be adjusted to dampen the strong echoes originating from the prosthetic valve.

THE AORTIC BALL PROSTHETIC VALVE

Valve Design

Many of the manufacturers that produce prosthetic heart valves offer at least one model of a ball prosthesis. Most of these consist of a suture ring and a ball occluder, a cage, either open at the ends or closed, and a ball made of silicon rubber or a hollow metal such as titanium. In some models, the struts or cage is covered with a fabric. The diameters of the ball range from 12 to 26 mm, and the ball excursions are from 7 to 11 mm. The suture ring diameters range from 19 to 40 mm (Fig. 12–20).

Anatomical Position

When a ball valve is placed in the aortic position, it is sutured into the aortic annulus with the struts protruding superiorly into the aorta. During ventricular systole, the valve opens as the ball moves superiorly and away from the valve orifice (Fig. 12–21).

Echocardiographic Appearance

A-Mode

On the A-mode, the aortic ball prosthesis appears as two heavy and distinct signals that represent the suture ring attachments to the anterior and posterior walls of the aortic root. Within these heavy echoes are two rapidly moving signals representing two sides of the ball as it passes in and out of the transducer beam in its opening and closing function (Fig. 12–22).

M-Mode

When placed in the aortic position, the ball valve is displayed on the M-mode as echoes within the aortic root that appear intermittently in correspondence with systole and diastole. Usually, the transducer beam will strike the valve as shown in Figure 12–21. During systole, if the valve is recorded from this angle, the echoes from the poppet will not move directly toward or away from the transducer beam but will produce slightly altered patterns. Usually, only minimal excursion is visualized and will be less than the maximum excursion of the valve (see Figure 12–22).

Because it is not readily possible to record the full excursion of the valve in the aortic position, any correlation between the measured excursion of the poppet and the analysis of prosthetic valve function is discouraged. It is possible, however, when serial echocardiograms are performed, to detect changes in the valve's overall pattern and to note the presence of increased echoes within the root or around the struts, which could represent thrombus or clot formation.

With some ball valves, the saw-toothed appearance commonly seen with the normal aortic valve cusps during systole is present (Fig. 12–23). This is thought to represent oscillations caused by the pressure being exerted through the aortic valve during systole.

A study by Johnson et al.[2] showed that poppets composed of different materials

Text continued on page 259

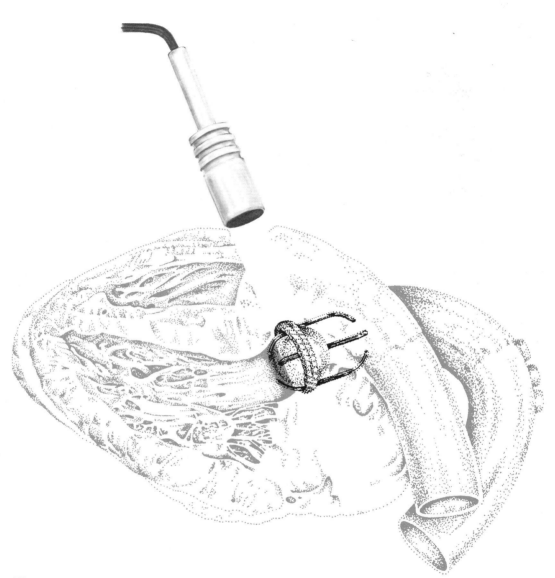

Figure 12–21.   A Smeloff-Cutter aortic prosthetic ball valve in the closed position. During systole, with the contraction of the left ventricle, the force of the ejected blood forces the ball to move superiorly. As a result, the ball passes in and out of the ultrasound beam with its opening and closing motion. (Smeloff-Cutter aortic prosthetic ball valve courtesy of Human Prosthetics, Cutter Laboratories, Inc.)

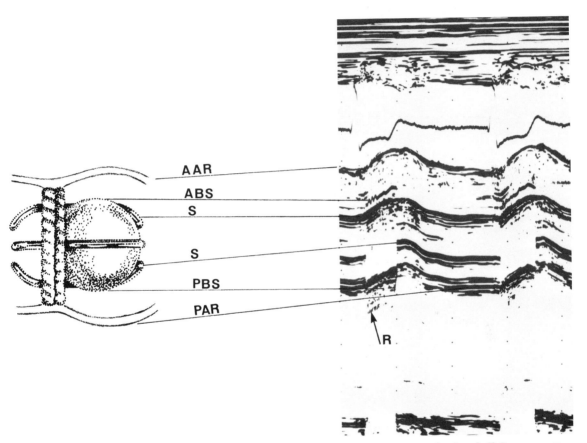

Figure 12–22. M-mode representation of the various component parts of a Smeloff-Cutter aortic valve (AAR = anterior aortic root wall; ABS = anterior ball surface; S = strut; PBS = posterior ball surface; PAR = posterior aortic root wall; R = reverberation echo [arrow]).

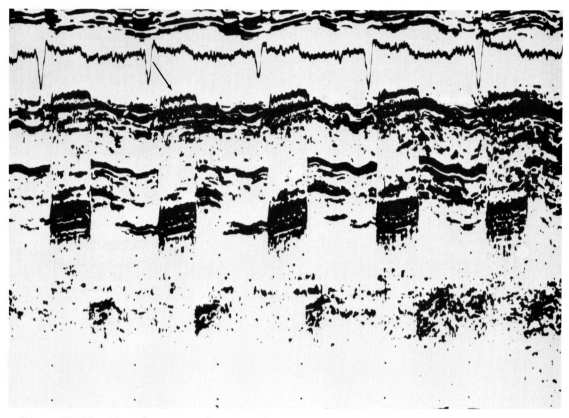

Figure 12–23.   M-mode tracing of a Starr-Edwards prosthesis in the aortic position. Note the saw-toothed appearance of the anterior ball surface during systole (arrow). These oscillations occur as a result of the pressure that is being exerted through the valve orifice.

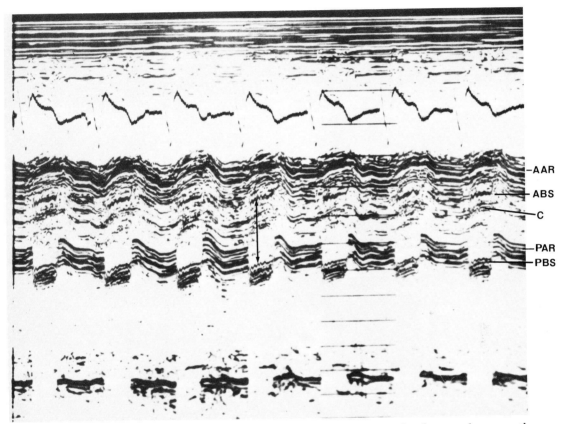

Figure 12-24.   M-mode tracing of a #3 Smeloff-Cutter prosthesis. The distance between the anterior ball surface and the posterior ball surface (arrow) measures approximately 2.4 cm. When multiplied by a conversion factor of 0.64, the result is 1.5 cm, which is the actual diameter of this size ball in the Cutter prosthesis. (AAR = anterior aortic root wall; ABS = anterior ball surface; C = cage; PAR = posterior aortic root; PBS = posterior ball surface).

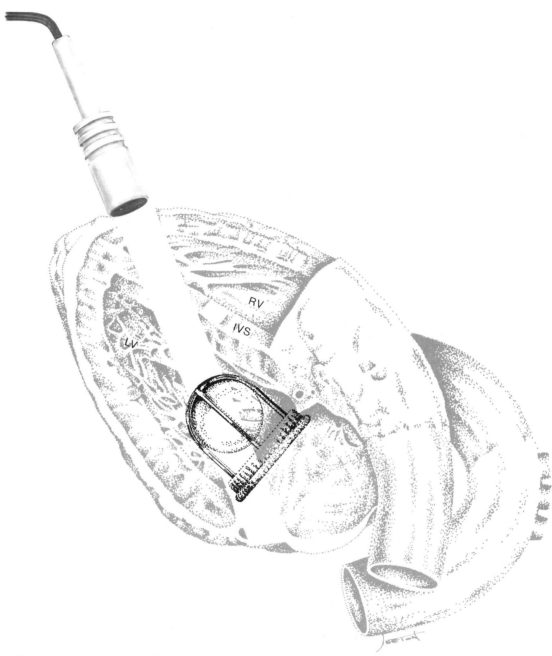

Figure 12–25. A Starr-Edwards ball valve in the mitral position. The poppet moves into the left ventricular cavity as blood is ejected through the mitral orifice and into the left ventricle. The transducer beam strikes the ball parallel to the long axis of its motion (RV = right ventricle; IVS = interventricular septum; LV = left ventricle). (Starr-Edwards ball valve courtesy of Edwards Laboratories, Division of American Hospital Supply.)

produced slightly different patterns on the echocardiogram. The results of an *in-vitro* study described in the same article showed that sound travels much slower through silicone rubber (960 mm/sec) than through tissue (1450 mm/sec). This difference accounts for the appearance of the posterior surface of the ball behind the suture ring in valves using a Silastic poppet. In order to determine the diameter of the silicone rubber ball from the echocardiographic recording, the thickness of the ball as shown by echocardiography was multiplied by a conversion factor of 0.64. As demonstrated in Figure 12–24, the ball diameter measures approximately 2.5 cm on the echocardiogram. When multiplied by the conversion factor of 0.64, the correct diameter is 1.6 cm, which is the accurate ball diameter for a small Starr-Edwards ball prosthesis.

The same study showed that when a hollow metal ball was used, sound was reflected off the anterior ball surface only and that echoes from the posterior surface of the ball were not seen.

THE MITRAL BALL PROSTHETIC VALVE

Anatomical Position

When the ball prosthesis is placed in the mitral position, it is sutured into the mitral annulus with the struts extending into the left ventricular cavity (Fig. 12–25).

Echocardiographic Appearance

A-Mode

When placed in the mitral position, the ball prosthesis appears on the A-mode as two parallel echoes. These two echoes are representative of the cage or struts and the suture ring moving subtly with the motion of the heart. Within the margins of the cage and suture ring, two separate parallel echoes representing the anterior and posterior sides of the ball will be seen. These echoes move anteriorly with diastole and posteriorly at the onset of systole and exhibit a rigid motion much like that of a severely stenotic mitral valve.

M-Mode

Immediately posterior to the echoes of the interventricular septum, the valve cage is represented as a continuous echo that exhibits a subtle anterior motion during systole and moves posteriorly in diastole. Posterior to the echo originating from the valve cage is the anterior surface of the ball, which moves sharply anteriorly during diastole and contacts the cage echo. With the

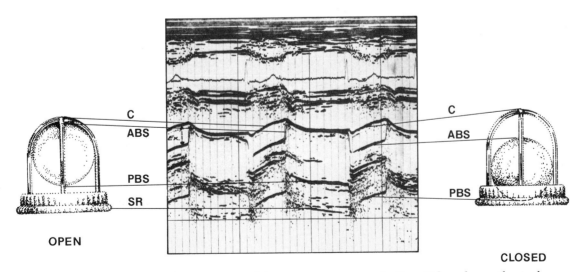

Figure 12–26. M-mode representation of the component parts of a Starr-Edwards prosthesis shown in the open and the closed positions. As the valve opens, the ball moves anteriorly toward the transducer (EX = ball excursion; C = cage; ABS = anterior ball surface; PBS = posterior ball surface; SR = suture ring). (Suture ring is not visualized on this tracing when the ball is in the closed position.)

QRS complex, at the onset of systole, the ball moves rapidly posteriorly to its closed position. The posterior side of the ball can be seen moving parallel to the anterior ball echo. Moving with much the same motion as the cage echoes is a band of thicker echoes representing the suture ring of the valve (Fig. 12–26). As previously discussed, the comparatively slower speed of sound through the Silastic ball gives the appearance of the ball in a position posterior to the suture ring.

Measuring the Mitral Ball Prosthesis

The maximum excursion of the poppet will vary with the type and size of valve used. With the Starr-Edwards prosthesis alone, the excursion can range from 7 to 11 mm. Knowing the size and the maximum excursion of the valve being recorded is of great value in analyzing its function. However, whether the poppet is opening completely or not can be determined without this knowledge. Transducer angulation is also critical in this evaluation. If the beam strikes the poppet from an angle that does not track its maximum excursion, it could appear that the valve is not opening completely. Careful observation of the valve during several cardiac cycles should indicate whether the poppet is converging tightly with the apex of the cage during diastole or if abnormally thickened echoes are pres-

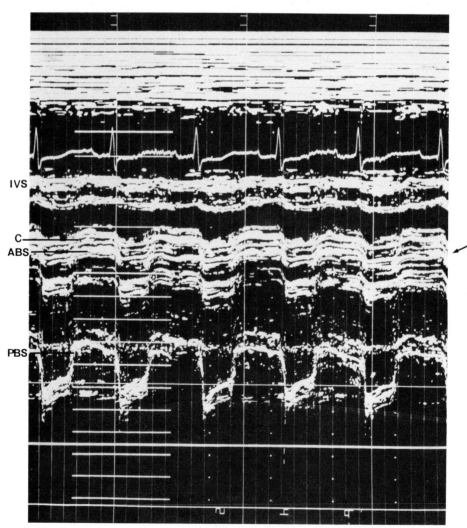

Figure 12–27.   M-mode tracing of a Starr-Edwards mitral valve prosthesis. The thickened band of echoes in the area of the anterior ball surface and cage represents clot formation (arrow). The presence of the clot formation was later confirmed on autopsy (IVS = interventricular septum; C = cage; ABS = anterior ball surface; PBS = posterior ball surface).

ent around the cage or suture ring (Fig. 12–27). Since the echoes originating from the posterior side of the ball and the suture ring cannot be seen to meet when the valve is closed, it would be very difficult to determine whether the poppet is closing completely without knowing the excursion of the valve in question.

CENTRAL FLOW VALVES

The central flow design artificial valve simulates some of the properties of the natural human valves. Since attempts to create synthetic valves of this type have been unsuccessful, the only central flow valves currently being used are composed of biological tissue.[7]

Autograft

An autograft valve is one taken from one anatomical position and grafted into another position in the same individual. Because it is almost identical to the aortic valve, the pulmonic valve may be used in the aortic position in an autograft replacement. The autograft valve is a completely viable transplant and therefore is capable of cellular regeneration. In most instances when the pulmonic autograft is performed, a homograft valve is used in the pulmonic position. Because of the relatively low pressure in the right ventricle, pulmonic replacement seems to be well-tolerated.

Homograft

A homograft is a valve taken from one individual for implantation in another individual. Presently, there are two types of homograft valves being used, fresh and preserved. Fresh homograft valves are collected under clean conditions and stored for use in a solution containing antibiotics. Viable cells have been found in these valves five years after implantation. Currently, these seem to be the most desired type of homograft valve.

Preserved valves are freeze-dried, and as a result, the viable cells are destroyed. Although initial results in the use of these valves were encouraging up to one year fol-

lowing implantation, a high percentage of patients developed murmurs of aortic incompetence.

Heterograft

A heterograft is a valve taken from an animal and implanted in a human. The most commonly used heterograft is a porcine valve (Fig. 12–28). Since these are nonviable prostheses, their function is dependent on maintenance of the elasticity in the natural valve.

Echocardiographic Appearance

Because it is similar to the natural aortic valve, the echocardiographic appearance of the central flow valve placed in the aortic position will also be similar on both the A-mode and the M-mode. The walls of the aortic root, however, may appear thicker than normal because a support ring is used with the valve. Clear visualization of the cusps of the valve is often difficult (Fig. 12–29).

When used in the mitral position, the porcine heterograft will appear between two heavy parallel echoes representing the anterior and posterior interfaces of the support ring. In a normally functioning heterograft valve, two of the cusps will be seen to sepa-

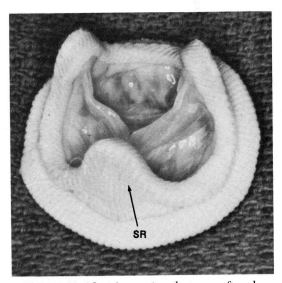

Figure 12–28. A porcine heterograft valve. The porcine valve is mounted in a support ring (SR) (arrow).

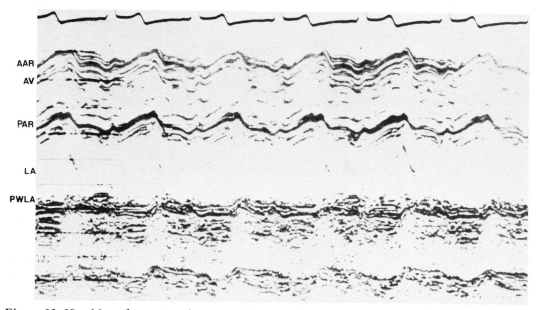

Figure 12–29. M-mode tracing of a porcine heterograft valve in the aortic position (AAR = anterior aortic root wall; AV = aortic valve; PAR = posterior aortic root wall; LA = left atrium; PWLA = posterior wall of the left atrium).

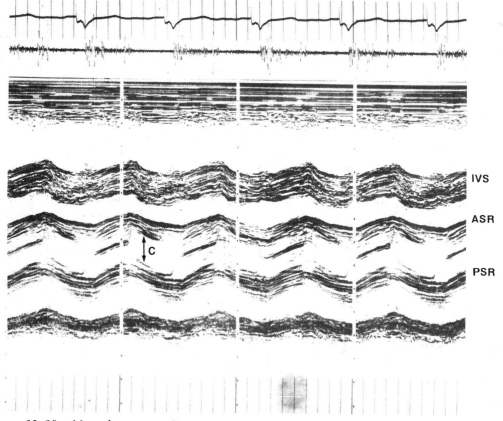

Figure 12–30. M-mode tracing of a porcine heterograft valve in the mitral position (IVS = interventricular septum; ASR = anterior support ring; C = cusps of the porcine valve; PSR = posterior support ring).

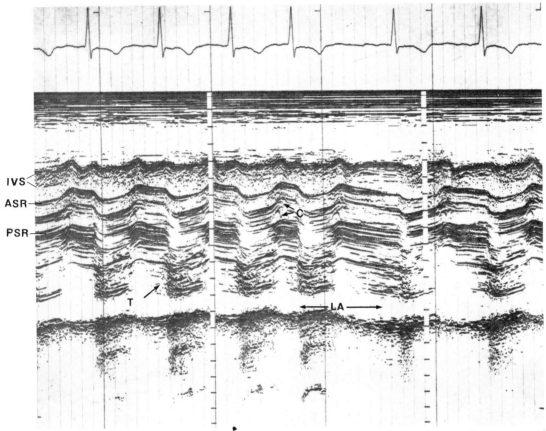

Figure 12–31. M-mode tracing of a Hancock porcine heterograft valve in the mitral position with thrombus formation present on the valve. Echoes representing the thrombus (T) are seen most prominently posterior to the support ring extending into the left atrium during systole. The opening of the valve cusps is not clearly visualized (IVS = interventricular septum; ASR = anterior support ring; C = valve cusps; PSR = posterior suture ring; LA = left atrium).

rate during diastole (Fig. 12–30). In optimal recordings, specific phases of opening will be seen that relate to those of the normal mitral valve. There is an initial opening of the cusps, partial closure, and then a reopening (A wave) coinciding with atrial systole.

Figure 12–31 is an M-mode tracing of a patient with a porcine heterograft valve in the mitral position. Excessive echoes are visualized posterior to the support ring and are most prominent during systole. These echoes represent clot formation present around the valve which extends through the valve and into the left atrium during systole (Fig. 12–31).

The echocardiographic appearance of calcific stenosis of a homograft valve in the mitral position has been described by Horowitz and associates.[7] In their study,

they described the calcification as a band of dense, heavy echoes seen within the margins of the two parallel echoes representative of the anterior and posterior support ring. Also noted was a decrease in the diastolic slope of the support echo, which was thought to suggest a reduced rate of ventricular filling.

REFERENCES

1. Ellis JL, Phillips B, Friedewald VE, and Diethrich EB: Evaluation of the Bjork-Shiley prosthetic valve by echocardiography. Ultrasound in Medicine 1:71, 1975.
2. Johnson ML, Patton B, and Holmes J: Ultrasonic evaluation of prosthetic valve motion. Circulation 41(Suppl II):3–9, 1970.
3. Bjork VO, and Olin C: A hydrodynamic comparison between the new tilting disc aortic valve prosthesis (Bjork-Shiley) and the corresponding prosthe-

ses of Starr-Edwards, Kay-Shiley, Smelloff-Cutter and Wada-Cutter in the pulse duplicator. Scand J Thor Cardiovasc Surg 4:31, 1970.

4. Alderman EL, Rytand D, Crow R, Finegan RE, and Harrison DC: Normal and prosthetic atrioventricular valve motion in atrial flutter. Correlation of ultrasound, vectorcardiographic and phonocardiographic findings. Circulation 45:1206, 1972.

5. Bjork VO, Book K, and Holmgren A: Significance of position and opening angle of the Bjork-Shiley tilting disc valve in mitral surgery. Scand J Thor Cardiovasc Surg 7:187, 1973.

6. Reid KG: Mitral valve action and the mode of ventricular filling. Nature 223:1383, 1969.

7. Horowitz MS, Goldman DJ, and Popp RL: Echocardiographic diagnosis of calcific stenosis of a stented aortic homograft in the mitral position. J Clin Ultrasound 2:179, 1974.

GLOSSARY OF CARDIAC TERMS

aneurysm — A spindle-shaped or sac-like bulging of the wall of a vein or artery caused either by weakening of the wall with disease or by an abnormality present at birth.

annulus — A small, ringlike supporting structure (usually used as "mitral valve annulus").

anterior — Referring to the frontal aspect of an organ; forward; antonym of posterior.

aorta — The main trunk artery, which receives blood from the left ventricle. It originates from the base of the heart, arches up over the heart like a cane handle, and passes down through the chest and abdomen in front of the spine. It branches off into many lesser arteries that conduct blood to all parts of the body except the lung. (See also *pulmonary circulation*.)

aortic arch — That segment of the aorta that curves up like the handle of a cane over the top of the heart.

aortic insufficiency — Defect in closure of the aortic valve that results in improper backflow into the left ventricle of blood delivered through the valve to the aorta.

aortic stenosis — Obstruction of aortic valve function caused by narrowing of or stricture of the aorta either slightly above or below the structure.

aortic valve — Valve at the junction of the aorta and the left ventricle. It is composed of three cup-shaped membranes called semilunar leaflets, which open to allow blood to flow from the left ventricle into the aorta and close to prevent backflow.

aortography — Radiographic visualization of the aorta and its major branches. This is made possible by the direct injection of radio-opaque dye into the aorta.

apex — The blunt, rounded end of the heart, directed downward, forward, and to the left.

arrhythmia — An abnormal rhythm of the heartbeat.

arterial blood — Oxygenated blood. The blood oxygenated in the lungs is passed to the left atrium via the pulmonary veins. It is then pumped by the left ventricle of the heart into the aorta, from which connecting arteries carry it to all parts of the body.

arteriosclerosis — Commonly called hardening of the arteries. This is a genetic term that includes a variety of conditions that cause the artery walls to become thick and hard, with reduced elasticity. (See also *atherosclerosis*.)

artery — A blood vessel that carries blood from the heart to the various parts of the body. All arteries carry oxygenated blood, except the pulmonary artery, which carries blood from the right heart to the lungs for oxygenation.

atherosclerosis — A kind of arteriosclerosis in which the inner layer of the artery wall is made thick and irregular by deposits of a fatty substance. These deposits (atheromata) project above the surface of the inner layer of the artery and thus decrease the diameter of the internal channel of the vessel.

atrial septum — Muscular wall separating left and right atria. (Sometimes called interatrial septum or interauricular septum.)

atrioventricular valves — Two valves located between the upper and lower chambers on either side of the heart. On the right side of the heart, the atrioventricular valve is called the tricuspid valve; on the left side, it is called the mitral valve.

atrium — One of the two upper chambers of the heart. Also called auricle, although this is now generally used to describe only the very tip of the atrium. The right atrium receives unoxygenated blood from the veins. The left atrium receives oxygenated blood from lungs. Capacity in the adult is approximately 57 cc.

auricle — Atrium.

auricular septum — Atrial septum.

auscultation — The act of listening to sounds within the body, usually with the aid of a stethoscope.

autonomic nervous system — Sometimes called the involuntary or vegetative nervous system. It controls tissues not under voluntary control, e.g., glands, heart, and smooth muscles.

bacterial endocarditis — An inflammation of the inner layer of the heart caused by bacteria. The lining of the heart valves is most frequently affected. Most commonly, this condition is a complication of an infectious disease, an operation, or an injury.

bicuspid valve — Having two cusps.

blood pressure — The pressure of the blood in the arteries. (1) *Systolic blood pressure.* Blood pressure when the heart muscle is contracted. (2) *Diastolic blood pressure.* Blood pressure when the heart muscle is relaxed between beats. Blood pressure is generally expressed by two numbers, as 120/80, with the first number representing the systolic pressure, and the second number, the diastolic pressure.

blue babies — Babies having a blueness of skin (cyanosis) caused by insufficient oxygen in the arterial blood. This often indicates a heart defect but may have other causes, such as premature birth or impaired respiration.

bradycardia — An abnormally slow heart rate. Generally, anything below 60 beats per minute is considered abnormal.

Beall (Bell) valve — A disc-type of prosthetic valve that is usually used in the mitral position.

capillaries — Extremely small blood vessels forming a network between the arterioles and the veins. The walls are composed of a single layer of cells through which oxygen and nutrients are carried.

cardiac — Pertaining to the heart.

cardiac catheterization — The introduction of a small-caliber catheter through a vein or artery directly into the heart to permit x-ray visualization of the cardiac chambers and the coronary arteries.

cardiac cycle — One total heartbeat, i.e., one complete contraction (systole) and relaxation (diastole) of the heart. In man, this normally occupies about 0.85 sec.

cardiac output — The amount of blood pumped by the heart every minute.

cardiovascular — Pertaining to the heart and blood vessels.

carditis — Inflammation of the heart.

carotid arteries — The left and right common carotid arteries are the principal arteries supplying blood to the head and neck. Each has two main branches, the external carotid artery and the internal carotid artery.

cerebral vascular accident — Impaired blood flow to some part of the brain, generally caused by (1) a blood clot forming in the vessel (cerebral thrombosis); (2) a rupture of the blood vessel wall (cerebral hemorrhage); (3) a piece of clot or other material from another part of the vascular system that flows to the brain and obstructs a cerebral vessel (cerebral embolism); or (4) pressure on a blood vessel, as by a tumor. Sometimes called "cerebrovascular accident," "apoplectic stroke," or simply "stroke."

cholesterol — A fat-like substance found in animal tissue. The normal level for Americans is assumed to be between 180 and 230 mg per 100 cc of blood. A higher level is often associated with high risk of coronary atherosclerosis.

chordae tendineae — Fibrous cords that serve as guy ropes to hold the valves between the upper and lower chambers of the heart secure when they are forced closed by pressure of blood in the lower chambers. The cords stretch from the cusps of the valves to the papillary muscles located in the walls of the lower heart chambers.

circulatory — Pertaining to the heart, blood vessels, and the circulation of the blood.

coarctation of the aorta — One of several congenital heart defects characterized by a pressing together, or a narrowing, of the aorta.

collateral circulation — circulation of the blood through a network of smaller blood vessels when a main vessel becomes obstructed.

commissurotomy — An operation to widen the opening in a heart valve that has become narrowed by scar tissue. The individual cusps of the valve are cut or spread apart along the natural line of their closure. This operation is often performed in cases of rheumatic heart disease.

congenital anomaly — An abnormality present at birth.

congestive heart failure — When the heart is unable to pump all the blood that returns to it, blood backs up in the veins leading to the heart. A congestion or accumulation of fluid in various parts of the body (lungs, legs, abdomen, and so on) may result from the heart's failure to maintain adequate circulation. (See also *myocardial insufficiency*.)

constrictive pericarditis — A shrinking and thickening of the outer sac of the heart, which impairs the normal contraction and expansion of the heart muscle.

coronary arteries— Two arteries arising from the aorta, arching down over the top of the heart, and bifurcating into several branches that spread to conduct blood to the heart muscle.

coronary atherosclerosis — Commonly called coronary heart disease. An irregular thickening of the inner layer of the walls of the arteries that conduct blood to the heart muscle. The internal channel of the coronary artery then becomes narrowed, and the blood supply to the heart muscle is reduced. (See also *atherosclerosis*.)

coronary occlusion — An obstruction (generally a blood clot) in a branch of one of the coronary arteries, which impedes the flow of blood to some part of the heart muscle. The affected area of the heart muscle then dies because of lack of blood supply. This tissue death is commonly known as a coronary heart attack or simply a heart attack. (See also *myocardial infarction*.)

coronary thrombosis — Formation of a clot in a branch of one of the coronary arteries. (See also *coronary occlusion*.)

cor pulmonale — Heart disease resulting from disease of the lungs or of the blood vessels in the lungs. This is due to resistance to the passage of blood through the lungs.

cusp — A leaflike flap that forms one of several segments of a cardiac valve.

cyanosis — Blueness of skin caused by insufficient oxygen in the blood. Oxygen is carried in the blood by hemoglobin, which is bright red when saturated with oxygen. When hemoglobin is not carrying oxygen, it is purple and is called reduced hemoglobin. The blueness of the skin occurs when the amount of hemoglobin reduction exceeds 5 gm per 100 cc of blood.

decompensation — Inability of the heart to maintain adequate circulation, usually resulting in a waterlogging of tissues. A person whose heart is failing to maintain normal circulation is said to be "decompensated."

dextrocardia — Two congenital phenomena involving positioning of the heart are often described as dextrocardia. The first is a condition in which the heart is slightly rotated and lies almost entirely in the right (instead of the left) side of the chest. The second is a condition in which there is a complete transposition, the left chambers of the heart being on the right side, and the right chambers on the left side, so that the heart presents a mirror image of the normal heart.

diastole — In the cardiac cycle, the period of relaxation of the heart. Auricular diastole is the period of relaxation of the atria; ventricular diastole, the period of relaxation of the ventricles.

digitalis — A drug derived from leaves of the foxglove plant. Serves to strengthen the contraction of the heart muscle, slow the rate of contraction of the heart, and by improving the efficiency of the heart, may promote the elimination of fluid from body tissues.

dilation — A stretching or enlargement of the heart or blood vessels.

diuresis — Increased excretion of urine.

ductus arteriosus — A small duct in the heart of the fetus between the artery leaving the left side of the heart (aorta) and the artery leaving the right side of the heart (pulmonary artery). Normally, this duct closes soon after birth. (See also *patent ductus arteriosus*.)

dyspnea — difficult or labored breathing.

edema — Swelling due to abnormally large amounts of fluid in the tissues of the body.

electrocardiogram (ECG, EKG) — A graphic recording of the electrical currents produced by the heart.

embolism — The blocking of a blood vessel by a clot or other substance carried in the blood stream.

embolus — A blood clot (or other substance such as air, fat, tumor) inside a blood vessel. (See also *thrombus*.)

endocarditis — Inflammation of the inner layer of the heart (endocardium) usually associated with acute rheumatic fever, bacteria, or some other infectious agent.

endocardium — A thin, smooth membrane forming the inner surface of the heart.

epicardium — The outer layer of the heart wall. Also called the visceral pericardium.

etiology — The sum of knowledge about the causes of a disease.

extrasystole — A contraction of the heart that occurs prematurely and interrupts the normal rhythm.

Fallot, Etienne Louis Arthur (1850–1911) — French physician who gave an important description of a congenital heart defect known as the tetralogy of Fallot. (See also *tetralogy of Fallot*.)

fibrillation — Uncoordinated contractions of the heart muscle occurring when the individual muscle fibers take up independent, irregular contractions.

fluoroscopy — The examination of a structure deep in the body by means of observing on a screen the display of fluorescence caused by x-rays transmitted through the body.

foramen ovale — An oval hole between the left and right upper chambers of the heart that normally closes shortly after birth. Its failure to close is the congenital defect known as patent foramen ovale.

hypercholesteremia — An excess of cholesterol in the blood. Sometimes called hypercholesterolemia or hypercholesterinemia. (See also *cholesterol*.)

hyperlipemia — An excess of fat or lipids in the blood.

hypertension — Commonly called high blood pressure. An unstable or persistent elevation of blood pressure above the normal range (100 mm Hg), which may eventually lead to increased heart size and kidney damage. (See also *primary hypertension* and *secondary hypertension*.)

hypertrophy — The enlargement of a tissue or organ due to increase in the size of its constituent cells. This may result from a demand for increased work.

hypoxia — Less than normal content of oxygen in the organs and tissues of the body. At very high altitudes, a healthy person suffers from hypoxia because of insufficient oxygen in the air that he breathes.

IHSS — Idiopathic hypertrophic subaortic stenosis. A condition characterized by asymmetric hypertrophy of the interventricular septum and consequent narrowing of the left ventricular outflow tract.

incompetent valve — Any valve that does not close tight, thus permitting backflow in the wrong direction. (See also *valvular insufficiency*.)

infarct — An area of tissue that is damaged or dies as a result of insufficient blood supply. Frequently used in the phrase "myocardial infarct," referring to damage to or death of an area of the heart muscle.

insufficiency — Incompetency. In the term "valvular insufficiency," an improper closing of the valves, which admits a backflow of blood in the wrong direction. In the term "myocardial insufficiency," inability of the heart muscle to do a normal pumping job.

interatrial septum — Atrial septum.

in vitro — Literally means "in glass," hence, in a laboratory vessel. Describes study of a phenomenon outside a living body under laboratory conditions.

in vivo — Describes study of a phenomenon within the living body.

ischemia — A local, usually temporary, deficiency of blood in some part of the body, often caused by a constriction or an obstruction of the blood vessel supplying that part.

lipid — Fat.

lipoprotein — A complex of fat and protein molecules.

mitral valve — The bicuspid cardiac valve located between the upper and lower chambers of the left side of the heart.

murmur — An abnormal heart sound, sounding like fluid passing an obstruction, heard between the normal "lub-dub" heart sounds.

myocardial infarction — The damaging or death of an area of the heart muscle resulting from a reduction in the blood supply delivered through the coronary arteries.

myocardial insufficiency — Inability of the heart muscle to maintain normal circulation. (See also *congestive heart failure.*)

myocarditis — Inflammation of the heart muscle.

myocardium — The muscular wall of the heart. The thickest of the three layers of the heart wall, it lies between the inner layer (endocardium) and the outer layer (epicardium).

nitroglycerin — A drug (one of the nitrates) that relaxes the muscles in the blood vessels. A vasodilator often used to relieve attacks of angina pectoris and spasm of the coronary arteries.

open-heart surgery — Cardiac surgery performed with the patient on cardiopulmonary bypass, a mechanical means of pumping and oxygenating blood. This mechanical substitution for heart and lungs permits direct operation on the heart or the coronary arteries.

organic heart disease — Heart disease caused by a structural abnormality of the heart or circulatory system.

pacemaker — The natural pacemaker of the heart consists of a small mass of specialized cells in the right upper chamber of the heart that give rise to the electrical impulses that initiate contractions of the heart. Also called sinoatrial node or S-A node of Keith-Flack. The term "pacemaker," or more correctly "electric cardiac pacemaker" or "electrical pacemaker," is applied to an electrical device implanted to substitute for a defective natural pacemaker and control the beating of the heart by a series of rhythmic electrical discharges. If the electrodes that deliver the discharges to the heart are placed outside the chest, the implanted device is termed an "external pacemaker." If the electrodes are placed within the chest wall, it is called an "internal pacemaker."

palpitation — A fluttering of the heart or an abnormal rate or rhythm of the heart experienced by the person himself.

pancarditis — Inflammation of the whole heart, including its inner layer (endocardium), the heart muscle (myocardium), and the outer sac (pericardium).

papillary muscles — Small bundles of muscles in the walls of the lower chambers of the heart to which the cords attached to the cusps of the valves (chordae tendineae) are connected. When the valves are closed, these muscles contract and tighten the cords to hold the valve cusps firmly shut.

paraplegia — Loss of both motion and sensation in the lower part of the body. Most commonly, this is due to damage to the spinal cord, but it sometimes results from a blood clot or hemorrhage in an artery conducting blood to the spinal cord.

parietal pericardium — A thin, membranous sac that surrounds the heart and the roots of the great vessels. The outer layer of the pericardium.

paroxysmal tachycardia — An episode of rapid heart action that begins and ends suddenly.

patent ductus arteriosus — A congenital heart defect in which a small duct between the aorta and the pulmonary artery, which normally closes soon after birth, remains open. Through this duct, blood from both sides of the heart is pumped into the pulmonary artery and into the lungs. This defect is sometimes called simply "patent ductus."

patent foramen ovale — A congenital heart defect in which an oval hole between the left and right atria, which normally closes shortly after birth, remains open.

pathology — The scientific study of the essential nature of disease and structural and functional changes it causes.

percussion — Tapping the body as an aid in diagnosing the condition of parts beneath by the sound obtained, much as one taps on a barrel to detect its fullness.

pericarditis — Inflammation of the thin, membranous sac (pericardium) that surrounds the heart.

pericardium — The thin, membranous sac that surrounds the heart and roots of the great vessels.

peripheral resistance — The resistance offered by the arterioles and the capillaries to the flow of blood from the arteries to the veins. An increase in peripheral resistance causes a rise in blood pressure.

primary hypertension — Sometimes called "essential hypertension" and commonly known as "high blood pressure." An elevated blood pressure not ascribable to kidney disease or other evident disorders.

propagation — Reproduction.

prophylaxis — Preventive treatment.

pulmonary artery — The large artery that conveys unoxygenated (venous) blood from the right ventricle to the lungs. This is the only artery that carries unoxygenated blood; all others circulate oxygenated blood throughout the body.

pulmonary circulation — The circulation of the blood through the lungs. Flow is initiated from the right ventricle, through the pulmonary artery, to the lungs. The oxygenated blood is then delivered from the lungs, through the pulmonary veins, to the left atrium. (See also *systemic circulation.*)

pulmonary hypertension — An increase of pressure within the pulmonary artery to above 30 mm Hg systolic and 12 mm Hg diastolic.

pulmonary stenosis — Narrowing of the opening into the pulmonary artery from the right ventricle.

pulmonary valve — The valve formed by three cup-shaped membranes at the junction of the pulmonary artery and the right ventricle. When the right ventricle contracts, the pulmonary valve opens, and blood is forced into the pulmonary artery. When the chamber relaxes, the valve closes to prevent a backflow of the blood.

pulmonary veins — Four veins (two from each lung) that conduct oxygenated blood from the lungs into the left atrium.

pulse — Arterial expansion and contraction that may be detected with the finger.

pulse pressure — The difference between the blood pressure in the arteries when the heart is in contraction (systole) and when it is in relaxation (diastole).

quinidine — A drug sometimes used to treat abnormal rhythms of the heartbeat.

regurgitation — The backward flow of blood through a defective valve.

renal circulation — The circulation of the blood through the kidneys. Important in heart disease because of its function in the elimination of water, chemical elements, and waste products from the body.

reserpine — One of the organic substances found in the root of the plant *Rauwolfia serpentina.* The drug lowers blood pressure, slows the heart rate, and has a sedative effect. It is an antihypertensive agent.

rheumatic fever — A disease, usually occurring in childhood, which may develop secondary to a streptococcal infection. It is characterized by one or more of the following: fever, sore, swollen joints, skin rash, involuntary twitching of the muscles (called chorea or St. Vitus Dance), and small nodes under the skin. In some cases the infection affects the heart and may result in scarring of the valves, weakening of the heart muscle, or damage to the pericardium.

S-A node — Sinoatrial node; Tissue located in the right atrium that generates electrical currents throughout the heart.

sclerosis — Hardening, usually due to an accumulation of fibrous tissue.

secondary hypertension — Elevated blood pressure secondary to specific diseases or infections.

semilunar valves — Cup-shaped valves. The aortic valve and the pulmonary valve are semilunar valves. They consist of three cup-shaped leaflets that open to allow passage of blood from one chamber to another and close to prevent backflow of blood.

septum — A dividing wall. (See also *atrial septum.*)

shunt — A passage between two blood vessels or an opening between the two sides of the heart. In surgery, the operation to form a passage between blood vessels to divert blood from one part of the body to another.

sinoatrial node — See *S-A node.*

sinuses of Valsalva — Three pouches in the wall of the aorta behind the three cup-shaped membranes of the aortic valve. The coronary arteries arise from this point on the aortic root. The sinuses of Valsalva have been designated according to the disposition of the coronary arteries to which they give rise. Thus, they are termed the right and left anterior sinuses and the posterior, or noncoronary, sinus.

stenosis — A narrowing or stricture of an opening. Chiefly, mitral stenosis and aortic stenosis, meaning that the valve has become narrowed and does not function normally.

stroke — (See *cerebral vascular accident.*)

stroke volume — The amount of blood pumped out of the heart with each contraction.

syncope — A faint. One cause for syncope can be an insufficient blood supply to the brain.

syndrome — A set of symptoms that occur together and are therefore given a name to indicate that particular combination.

systemic circulation — The circulation of the blood through all parts of the body except the lungs, the flow being from the left ventricle, through the body, to the right atrium. (See also *pulmonary circulation.*)

systole — In each cardiac cycle, the period of contraction of the heart. Atrial systole is the period of the contraction of the upper chambers of the heart. Ventricular systole is the period of the contraction of the lower chambers of the heart.

tachycardia — An abnormally fast heart rate, generally over 100 beats per minute.

tetralogy of Fallot — A congenital malformation of the heart involving four distinct defects (hence tetralogy). Named for Etienne Fallot, the French physician who described the condition in 1888. The four defects are:

1. An abnormal opening in the wall between the lower chambers of the heart.
2. Misplacement of the aorta, "over-riding" the abnormal opening, so that it receives blood from both the right and left lower chambers instead of only the left.
3. Narrowing of the pulmonary artery.
4. Enlargement of the right lower chamber of the heart.

thrombosis — The formation or presence of a blood clot (thrombus) inside a blood vessel or cavity of the heart.

thrombus — A blood clot that forms inside a blood vessel or cavity of the heart. (See also *embolus*.)

toxemia — The condition caused by poisonous substances in the blood.

toxic — Pertaining to poison.

tricuspid valve — A valve consisting of three cusps or triangular segments located between the upper and lower chambers in the right side of the heart. Its position corresponds to the mitral valve in the left side of the heart.

truncus arteriosus — Common aorta and pulmonary artery.

valvular insufficiency — The circulatory condition caused by valves that close improperly and allow a backflow of blood. (See also *incompetent valve*.)

vein — Any one of a series of vessels of the vascular system that carries blood from various parts of the body back to the heart. All veins conduct unoxygenated blood, except the pulmonary veins, which carry oxygenated blood from the lungs back to the heart.

INDEX

Page numbers in *italics* refer to illustrations.